Medical Imaging and Philosophy
Edited by Heiner Fangerau, Rethy Chhem, Irmgard Müller
and Shih-Chang Wang

KULTUR ANAMNESEN

Schriften zur Geschichte und Philosophie der Medizin und der Naturwissenschaften

Herausgegeben von Heiner Fangerau, Renate Breuninger und Igor Polianski

in Verbindung mit dem Institut für Geschichte, Theorie und Ethik der Medizin, dem Humboldt-Studienzentrum für Philosophie und Geisteswissenschaften und dem Zentrum Medizin und Gesellschaft der Universität Ulm

Band 3

Medical Imaging and Philosophy

Challenges, reflections and actions

Conference Proceedings

EDITED BY HEINER FANGERAU, RETHY CHHEM,
IRMGARD MÜLLER AND SHIH-CHANG WANG

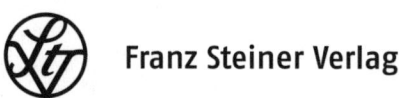 Franz Steiner Verlag

Umschlagabbildungen:
Reihenlogo: Walter Draesner, „Der Tod und der Anatom", Graphiksammlung „Mensch und Tod"
der Heinrich-Heine-Universität Düsseldorf
Abbildung: Paul Flechsig, Monatsschrift für Psychiatrie und Neurologie 26 (Suppl.1): I–IV (1909)

Bibliografische Information der Deutschen Nationalbibliothek:
Die Deutsche Nationalbibliothek verzeichnet diese Publikation in der Deutschen
Nationalbibliografie; detaillierte bibliografische Daten sind im Internet über
<http://dnb.d-nb.de> abrufbar.

© Franz Steiner Verlag, Stuttgart 2012
Druck: Laupp & Göbel, Nehren
Gedruckt auf säurefreiem, alterungsbeständigem Papier.
Printed in Germany.
ISBN 978-3-515-10046-5

INHALTSVERZEICHNIS

FOREWORD: MEDICAL IMAGING:
CHALLENGES, REFLECTIONS AND ACTIONS

Rethy Chhem, Heiner Fangerau, Irmgard Müller, Shih-chang Wang

Medical Imaging plays a prominent role in contemporary medical research and practice. At the same time imaging in its broadest sense, including illustration, diagramming, model-making, photography and other forms of image rendering, has a long tradition in medicine.

Imaging has served different purposes ranging from depicting to backing concepts or creating convincing evidence. Thus, imaging the human body has different aspects not only related to techniques or current interpretations of visual representations through medical imaging technologies. Furthermore, the way the human body was and is displayed in images also reflects a range of cultural, historical, artistic and scientific concerns.

Therefore, the editors of this book organized an international interdisciplinary conference in 2010 to bring together perspectives on Medical Imaging from medicine, philosophy, history and arts. The aim of the conference was to discuss medical images as scientific representations, their inherent ontologies and ethical aspects related to representing the human body.

The topics that were discussed included the production of knowledge using imaging techniques and the commonality of that knowledge across imaging modalities, the role of data and data collection for medical diagnosis and communication, the role of formal ontologies in representation and communication with medical images, norms of health and disease and the understanding of body (and mind) as they are shaped by imaging technologies, and the interdependence of technology, medicine and information science.

Now we are proud to present with this book the proceedings of this interdisciplinary conference including representative examples of what was presented and discussed. We will start with two papers by Rethy Chhem and Shih-chang Wang reflecting on Medical Imaging from the perspective of medicine and radiology. We will then delve into questions of representing ontologies and "scientific truth" with the help of images. The papers by Irmgard Müller and Heiner Fangerau, James Overton and Cesare Romagnoli, Kirsten Brukamp, Frederick Gilbert and Heiner Fangerau and Robert Lindenberg examine the evidentiary status of images, ontological structures in radiology, processing procedures, brain reading metaphors and chains of representation in medical imaging. This more epistemologically oriented section is followed by a section focusing practices and media in imaging the body. Fabio Zampieri, Alberto Zanatta and Maurizio Rippa Bonati reflect upon Iconography and Wax models in the promotion of vaccination Katsiaryna Laryionava examines how contemporary art redefines the human body, Richard Hoppe-Sailer,

Rainer-M. E. Jacobi and Sarah Sandfort critically analyse the interconnections between the spheres of visual representations, the body and knowledge and Kathrin Friedrich displays how the practices of a "sight collective" influence diagnostic procedures in computed tomography. In a final section Santiago Sia is "looking behind the image" and is raising in an outlook philosophical and ethical issues in medical imaging that might be in the focus of a following conference.

We hope that these conference proceedings with their wide scope are stimulating to readers interested in the status of medical images and their interpretation by different disciplines and that this book fosters further discussions. We wish to express our gratefulness to all the authors for their participation and to the German Research Foundation and the Centre for Medicine & Society, Ulm University for generously funding the publication of these conference proceedings.

The editors, July 2011

I. MEDICAL PERSPECTIVES –
USE AND REFLECTION

MEDICAL IMAGE: IMAGING OR IMAGINING?

Rethy K Chhem

INTRODUCTION

The rapid developments and progresses in medical imaging in the last three decades have radically improved and transformed the way physicians perceive and see the human body. These changes have totally revolutionized medical practice. Many organs and structures, which were in the past invisible to conventional X-ray examinations, are now revealed through sophisticated imaging modalities such as computed tomography (CT), ultrasound (US) or magnetic resonance imaging (MRI). Furthermore, nuclear imaging such as positron emission tomography (PET), is used together with CT or MRI to form "hybrid imaging" (i. e. PET/CT, PET/MRI) and enables a simultaneous study of both structure and function (or dysfunction). The pace and scope of such scientific and technologic progresses have brought a new paradigm to the generation of new knowledge, and resulted in a range of philosophical questions in both epistemic and ethical issues. In this paper, the reflection will focus mainly on these epistemological issues relating to the formation of medical images, which now play a pivotal role in medical decision-making. For examples, such issues are applicable to the diagnosis and therapy in cancer care: i. e. X-rays and MRI are used not only to detect a bone tumour, but also to establish its extension to the surrounding tissues, or to exclude metastasis from its original site to the distant organs such as the lungs or brain.

MEDICAL IMAGE: THE HISTORICAL PERSPECTIVE

The historical roots of this quest to look at the inside of the human body can be found in the ancient story of the Buddhist doctor, Jivaka who was known as "The legend of Jivaka and the King of Physician's tree". Jivika was a physician in the royal court of King Bimbisara (558 BC–491 BC) of Maghada in Ancient India, a thousand years ago. One day, outside the royal palace, Jivaka met a boy carrying a bundle of wood sticks on his back. Jivaka was surprised that he could see the boy's internal organs through his body. He recalled the magical property of the King-Doctor's tree, which would make the inside of the body visible. Jivaka bought the wood sticks from the boy, who then dropped the bundle to the ground. Suddenly, the intense light that illuminated the boy's internal organs faded away and his body returned back to normal. Jivaka pursued an "experiment" by applying each one of these sticks to the boy in turn until he has found the famous King-Doctor's wood stick. Jivaka kept this stick as a diagnostic tool for his medical practice (De Saint

Firmin 1916). This may be be the origin of the "ultrasound probe" as dreamed of by many other doctors of the ancient Buddhist kingdoms of Asia.

In Europe, until the 17th and 18th centuries, a doctor remained "at a distance" from a patient, because visual inspection alone seemed to be the most appropriate way to establish a diagnosis. By the end of the 18th century, this "clinical gap" was reduced as a result of the development of new clinical tools (Foucault 1989: 167), e.g. the auscultation of lungs and heart with a stethoscope. Because there is no disease without a seat (i.e. the origin of the disease), a closer "gaze" is necessary to establish a diagnosis. It was Giovanni Battista Morgagni from the University of Padua, who pioneered this approach, when he published his seminal work in 1761, on the "The seats and causes of diseases". While the distance between physician and patient was bridged by auscultation in the early 19th century, the pre-auscultation "clinical gap" was restored through medical imaging when radiologist assessed a patient "at a distance" using X-rays examination.

The process as described by Foucault by studying the body from the "symptomatic surface" to the "tissue surface" through the dissection of corpses (Foucault 1989: 166) was no longer necessary following the emergence of medical imaging, which started with the discovery of X-rays by Roentgen in 1896. The internal organs (the subject) are now "visible" by medical imaging. The Foucauldian "medical gaze" from the anatomo-clinical dimension (i.e. the surface of the human body) to a pathological anatomy dimension (i.e. the internal organ as the seat of disease) no longer requires an opening of the body. X-rays, ultrasound, magnetic fields and radio-frequency waves have replaced the scalpel. The invisible part of the human body is now revealed with great details through medical imaging.

MEDICAL IMAGE: THE PRODUCTION LINE

Modern medical imaging allows us to study the inside of the body. However, the many complex mathematical and technical processes for image acquisition and manipulation could lead to the generation of other signals, which do not seem (at least a priori) to be a reliable representation of the specimen. Such signals are called "artefacts". These artefacts could lead to interpretation errors and could increase the risk of making a wrong diagnosis. However, in other situations, these "artefacts" may in fact contribute to diagnosis, e.g. by delineating a blurred anatomical boundary between a tendon and the surrounding fatty tissues, i.e. the "anisotropic artefact" for an ultrasound procedure.

The key question is: "Does the image displayed on the monitor accurately represent reality, e.g. does this truly reflect the structures of a patient's knee in the MRI room"? The image displayed is the result of an interaction between an X-ray beam or an electro-magnetic and radiofrequency wave and the body. More recently, PET/ CT (Positron Emission Tomography/Computed Tomography) was introduced to clinical practice as a major tool for cancer imaging. This innovative technology allows not only an accurate delineation of anatomy, but also an assessment of an organ's functional and metabolic pattern. A radio-active tracer is injected intravenously before scanning. An image is obtained following a number of complex steps. To quote Dr. Vibhu Kapoor, "PET provides images of quantitative uptake of the radionuclide injected .... However, for accurate results, the images must be corrected for the effects of attenuation of the 511-keV photons as they pass through the patient. In contrast to PET, which used an external radioactive transmission scan, PET-CT uses CT transmission data to correct for attenuation differences. After reconstruction, the CT, attenuation-corrected, and attenuation-uncorrected images obtained from the unified PET and CT protocol are transferred to, integrated at, and displayed on the syngo software platform. Differential PET to CT weighting, crosshairs linking of the axial, coronal, and sagittal reformatted images, and interactive viewing of the CT, PET, and fused images are possible" (Kapoor et al, 2004). This lengthy excerpt from an article published in the radiology literature was selected purposely to show the complex process of image generation for a PET/CT procedure. The image is produced through a series of physical processes, which involve mathematical transformations and complex computations.

The black and white image obtained is conventionally "displayed" as a variation of tissue densities (CT), signal intensities (MRI) or echogenicity (ultrasound). To make this "scientific image" to resemble closer to the actual knee, computer programs enable the manipulations of cross-sectional 2-D images into a volumetric image. This is "post-processing", i.e. processing after the data set was acquired. The result is a "3-D reconstruction" of the 2-D images. This terminology sheds light on this new paradigm in the "visualization" of the human body, which clearly implies that such image is artificially created as a "scientific representation" of the body part being examined. The next step in this quest towards a more realistic image, with a closer resemblance to the original, is to process the data set by "virtual reality". However, the term "image" must be firstly defined. How "real" is this image when compared to the body part being examined? After all, the final image is the result of numerous image processing steps!

MEDICAL IMAGE: THE DEFINITIONS

Before discussing "medical image" further, it is important defining the term first. According to the Cambridge International Dictionary of English, an image is a "picture that is formed by a mirror or a lens" (1995: 704), or a "picture in the mind of what something or someone is like". This is far from how doctors define a medical image. The definition given by the French dictionary, "Le Petit Robert", is much closer to what we conceive as a medical image; i.e. a "representation of an object by graphic or plastic arts" (Le Petit Robert 1990: 960), which can be applied to the representation of an object by a "radiological process".

Of course, a medical image differs from a traditional painting. The latter is used by an artist to "communicate" his perception of an object through a drawing. Medical images are also construed, but in such case these "paintings" were generated, not by an artist, but by mathematical and physical processes. By this definition, a CT scan of the brain is a digital representation (CT image) of the brain (object).

A range of media is used to display these images, e. g. by films or workstation monitor. By extending this concept, a technique that allows the generation of images by using different types of radiation is called medical imaging (Le Petit Robert 1990: 961). The immense progress in medical imaging science and technology has provided scientists and physicians with a myriad of new ways to visualize the inside of the body and to evaluate both normal and abnormal internal organs. These advances raise a few original epistemic questions. For example, the images have become the centre of physicians' attention, who have requested imaging to identify the internal seat of disease. This leads to a kind of "image worship" of what Crowe referred to as the "icon of medicine" (Crowe 2008: 1627–1630). The patient's body part is displaced behind such construed medical images on which the medical gaze is now focused. Each radiologist should look beyond the image itself, as behind each set of images, there is a patient! It would be of interest to reflect on Plato's cave allegory in which the philosopher believed that those who would find freedom from the cave would only be those who understand that the shadows do not constitute reality. What then is the link between the patient's body part and the image displayed on the monitor? Do the MRI or CT images alone provide sufficient information to achieve a diagnosis? For example, when a radiologist identifies a mass on a CT scan, he then uses his knowledge and clinical judgement to raise the possibility of a tumour. Indeed, such medical imaging-based diagnosis must be confirmed by biopsy and histology of the specimen obtained.

How do these medical images, as a representation of the body, contribute to medical reasoning and judgments in the context of clinical practice? For instance, how can an image that is only a representation of a body part carry any value in the decision-making, which will affect a patient's welfare? These philosophical questions are even more relevant considering the current developments in medical imaging technology. These have reached a level of complexity and sophistication that have revolutionized digital images display on PACS (Pictures Archiving and Communication System) workstations, leading to a new paradigm of image interpretation.

In the late 1970s, a CT scan of the brain produced a dozen of images, while a current CT scan generates thousand of images, making the interpretation very challenging due to the large number of images to be reviewed. Furthermore, the increased complexity from all these technological advances in medical imaging has created an imperative to design computer-assisted diagnostic (CAD) systems and new image display strategies to assist radiologists in their diagnostic task in the future. (Jacobson 2006).

How accurate is the image a representation of the patient? How reliable is the medical image when it is used as a basis for important clinical decision-making? Are we imaging or imagining? As Dyson said, "blind men imagine what they don't see". (Dyson, in Lightman 2005: 254). Both radiologists and theoretical physicists are on the same deep enquiry journey: "seeing the unseen" to quote Dyson. During my two-decade tenure in academic radiology departments, I used to tease my trainees on whether they were "doing imaging" or "imagining" when I taught them the systematic analysis of medical images for diagnostic purpose. This central philosophical question about medical image, with a special focus on neuroscience, was addressed by Illes and Racine (2005).

MEDICAL IMAGE: THE "THINKING TOOL"

For centuries, images were used extensively in scientific representations and therefore serve as a tool for thinking. In the 15th century, the iconic genius Leonardo da Vinci, through his artistic and "scientific" work, has extensively used drawings and diagrams to illustrate the morphology and functions of man and nature (Cremante 2010). His innumerable experiments were probably the best examples of "scientific research" long before that methodology was recognized several centuries later. Physicists and mathematicians generally used equations to explain theories or concepts relating to the physical world. Indeed, in some situations, they used diagrams instead to clarify their thoughts or explain abstract concepts. Dirac explained complex and abstract mathematical concepts in quantum mechanics by projective geometry, a skill previously acquired when he was encouraged to develop "visual imagination" in art and drawing classes (Farmelo 2010: 130). Feynman, who was awarded the Nobel Prize in Physics in 1965, used pictorial diagrams instead of mathematical equations not only to describe quantum processes but also an innovative way to understand nature. This pictorial view of nature, which he called the "space-time approach", became a working language for particle physicists around the world (Dyson 2006: 271). Faraday reasoned and constructed his electromagnetic field concept by using schematic lines of force surrounding a magnetic bar (Nersessian 1992). In contrast to most mathematicians and physicists, natural historians of the 17th, 18th and 19th centuries and biologists of the 20th century often acquired knowledge and developed concepts by using pictures and diagrams. Their scientific knowledge was based on illustrations as they thought by visualizing. Imagination and visual thinking were also important in the development of chemistry (Rocke 2010). An excellent example is the use of a drawing to illustrate and explain the molecular structure of nucleic acids as proposed by Watson and Crick (1953). The historical and philosophical values of art in the creation of scientific knowledge have now been addressed actively by numerous scholars (Baigrie 1996). When images are used as a scientific representation in physics, natural history or medicine, they play a dual role. The first is to serve as a model for reasoning, i.e. a "thinking tool", to clarify or establish an emerging theoretical concept, which will lead to the building of new knowledge. The second is to teach a well-established scientific concept by promoting the dissemination of that knowledge.

An example in medical education for this latter role is in the teaching of anatomy to medical students. For the last several decades, anatomy dissection sessions have decreased significantly in medical education programmes (Older 2004). Students now learn human anatomy via web-based courses, cross sectional pictures from medical imaging databases, or models generated from CT images (Marker 2010; Wanibuchi 2010). For these students, who have no or limited dissection exposure, learning through the electronic media may distort the reality of human anatomy. This is a typical situation where "imaging" is transformed into "imagining" as a study of an object (human body) is actually a perception of an image obtained through a chain of man-made processes starting from the interaction of an X-ray beam with matter (human body) and finishing with the re-constructed images. This learning situation illustrates how future physicians will build knowledge: from a set of re-constructed medical images, instead of cadaver dissection-based teaching. On the other hand, one may also argue how a cadaver can reliably represent the true anatomy of a live individual. The key epistemic issue in medical imaging is that knowledge will be built from the study of an image of an object rather than from the observation of the object directly.

Leonardo da Vinci (1452–1519) is probably the best example of an artist and "scientist" who has used images, drawings and diagrams widely to build and disseminate knowledge. For Leonardo, "All our knowledge has its origin in our perception" (Richter 2008: 6). Observations through numerous experiments laid the foundation for this epistemological approach (Richter 2008: 10). Knowledge is gained through the senses, especially by visualization, for Leonardo. For that renaissance iconic polymath, observation and experience were far more important than theories in books" (Cremante 2010: 574). Two centuries later, John Locke (1632–1704) and subsequently David Hume (1711–1776) underwent a systematic study of epistemology that would become known as "empiricism" (Locke 1996; Hume 2008). Both philosophers claimed that knowledge was initially established by perception. Hence for Locke, "Tis no matter how things are: so the man observes but the agreement of his own observations, and talk comfortably, it is all truth, all certainty" (Locke 1996: 250). Along the same line of thinking, Hume firmly believes that "men learned from experience" (Hume 2008: 76). An empiricist's approach can be applied to the epistemological process in medical imaging where the radiologist would observe and study the image on the X-rays film or monitor and process this information before arriving at a most likely diagnosis. A radiologist could see through the body by using imaging equipment (X-rays, Ultrasound, CT or MRI) while Leonardo used his naked eyes to observe the internal organ of a human body by dissection.

The theory of knowledge as proposed by British empiricists like Hume and Locke sharply contrasted sharply to that proposed by rationalist philosophers like Rene Descartes (1596–1650) who argued that mental reasoning is more powerful to establish reliable knowledge than by using the senses. Reasoning must prevails over perception (Descartes 1950). For Descartes, real knowledge cannot be established either by senses alone, in particular by the eyes, or by pure imagination, i. e. "to form a mental picture" (Cambridge 1995); but only by a cautious process of mental reasoning. For example, Descartes saw "a number coats and hats moving through the street" when he looked out of a window. It was by reasoning Descartes come to the conclusion that there were actually people (not seen), wearing hats and coats while moving around. Indeed Descartes opposed to empiricism because as a mathematician, he believed objectivity could only be achieved through the use of rational thinking. Also as a dualist, mind and body are distinct and separated.

In modern clinical practice, medical imaging plays an increasing role in decision-making, for both diagnostic and therapeutic purposes. It is reasonable to ask whether medical imaging is an "imaging" or "imagining" process from an epistemological dimension. For me, medical imaging includes and relies on the following processes: the appropriate acquisition of images by the machine, the reliable perception of the images by the eyes of the radiologist, and the accurate interpretation of the images by the radiologist. Once these images have reached the brain and the mind of the radiologist, he or she will "imagine", i.e. form a mental image of the organ that he or she has learned from past anatomy courses. This mental process will project the image within the clinical context, after taking into consideration of the clinical symptoms and the results of laboratory tests. This evaluation by the assimilation of these data (medical images, clinical symptoms and biological results) requires some imaginative skills. Based on the deduction, these data will be considered as normal or abnormal. If abnormal, a most likely diagnosis will be selected from a gamut of diseases that share similar findings. Hence I would argue that medical imaging in clinical setting is a combination of both "imaging" and "imagining".

The widespread use of images as a "thinking tool" to establish knowledge leads to multiple ethical issues. Indeed, given the complexity of medical image re-construction and the other questions of accuracy and reality, one can ask what are the ethical issues faced by doctors when they use these images as a basis for important decision-making in daily practice. These ethical issues, although essential to the good practice of medicine, are beyond the scope of this paper.

In essence, lying behind every medical image is a patient. So let's look beyond these medical images!

ACKNOWLEDGEMENTS

I wish to thank Professor Santiago Sia, Dr James Overton and Dr Lawrence Lau for their valuable comments and suggestions.

REFERENCES

Baigrie, B. S. (1996) Picturing Knowledge: Historical and Philosophical Problems Concerning the Use of Art in Science. Toronto, University of Toronto Press,

Cambridge (1995), International Dictionary of English. Cambridge, Cambridge University Press

Cremante, S. (2010) Leonardo da Vinci. The complete works. Cincinnati, David & Charles Book

Crowe, J. K. (2008) Radiology: Icon of Medicine, Avatar of Change. AJR; 191: 1627–1630

De Saint Firmin, L. (1916) Médecine et légendes bouddhiques de l'Inde. Paris, Ernest Leroux, pp 30–31

Descartes, R. (1950) Textes choisies de Descartes. Tome Premier: Métaphysique et Physique. Classiques Garnier. Paris, Librairie Garnier Frères pp. 97–99

Dyson, F. (2006) The Scientist as Rebel. New York, New York Review Books

Farmelo, G. (2010) The Strangest Man: The Hidden Life of Paul Dirac, Quantum Genius. London, Faber and Faber

Foucault, M. (1989) The Birth of the Clinic: An Archaeology of Medical Perception. London, Routledge

Hume, D. (2008) An Enquiry Concerning Human Understanding. Oxford, Oxford University Press. (First published in 1748)

Illes J, Racine E. Imaging or imagining? A neuroethics challenge informed by genetics. Am J Bioeth. 2005 Spring;5(2):5–18.

Jacobson, F. L., Berlanstein, B. P., Andriole, K. P. (2006) Paradigm of Perception in Clinical Practice. J Am Coll Radiol, 3, 441–446

Kapoor, V., McCook, B., Torok, F. (2004) An Introduction to PET-CT Imaging. RadioGraphics, March (24), 523–543

Le Petit Robert (1990) Paris Dictionnaires Le Robert

Lightman A. (2005) A Sense of the Mysterious: Science and the Human Spirit. – New York, Pantheon Books

Locke, J. (1996) An essay concerning human understanding. Cambridge, Hackett Publishing Company. (First published in 1689)

Locke, J., Berkeley G., Hume, G., (1974) The empiricists. New York, Anchor Books

Marker, D. R., Bansal, A. K., Juluru, K., Magid, D. (2010) Developing a radiology-based teaching approach for gross anatomy in the digital era. Acad Radiol. Aug;17 (8): 1057–65

Morgagni, Giambattista. (1761) De Causis et Sedibus Morborum per anatomen indagatis. Venice: libri quinque, Remondini

Nersessian, N. (1992) How do scientists think? Capturing the dynamics of conceptual change in science. In Giere RN (ed.). *Cognitive models in science*. University of Minneapolis Press, 3–45

Older J. (2004) Anatomy: A Must for Teaching the Next Generation. Surgeon. Apr;2(2): 79–90

Richter, I. (2008) Leonardo da Vinci. Notebooks. Oxford, Oxford University Press

Rocke, A. J. (2010) Image and reality: Kekule, Kopp and the scientific imagination. Chicago, University of Chicago Press

Wanibuchi, M, Ohtaki, M., Fukushima, T., Friedman, A. H., Houkin, K. (2010) Skull base training and education using an artificial skull model created by selective laser sintering. Acta Neurochir. 152(6): 1055–59

Watson, J. D., Crick, F. H. C. (1953) A structure for deoxyribose nucleic acid. *Nature* 171, 737–738

PHILOSOPHICAL ASPECTS OF MEDICAL IMAGING FROM A RADIOLOGIST'S PERSPECTIVE

Shih-chang (Ming) Wang

ABSTRACT

We live in an age of extraordinary and stunningly rapid advances in medical imaging. Barely more than a century after the discovery of x-rays and radioactivity, we are using medical imaging to explore the human body in health and disease in ways that were unimaginable even 20 years ago. The extensive permeation of imaging into the practice of modern medicine has meant that much of medical practice has become dependent on it, almost like a habit-forming drug.

This chapter enumerates the various types of medical imaging technologies currently in widespread usage, highlights the strengths and limitations of these technologies, and hopefully will explain how radiologists and other imaging specialists use such technologies to make diagnoses and thus influence or guide the treatment of patients. It explores the nature of radiological expertise, the process of imaging-based diagnostic decision-making, and raises the need for philosophical understanding in medical imaging today.

MEDICAL IMAGING AND PHILOSOPHY

Imaging has a unique place in modern clinical medicine. It is at the intersection of engineering, physics, chemistry, biology, anatomy, medicine, surgery, pharmacology and physiology. After a relatively leisurely start in the first half of the 20th century, today it is advancing and expanding at a breathtaking pace. Since the discovery of x-rays by Röntgen (Röntgen 1895), medical imaging has revolutionized our understanding of the normal human body and the manner in which disease affects its structure, function and physiology. X-ray devices were rapidly developed for clinical application and their use spread across the globe in an unprecedented and extraordinarily rapid fashion. For the first time it was possible to see inside the human body without incising the skin. The field of clinical radiology emerged within 5 years of Roentgen's discovery, and was solely dependent on various uses of x-rays for over 50 years until the advent of newer imaging modalities in the second half of the 20th century.

The rapid development and clinical application of several new imaging technologies has, in conjunction with x-rays, transformed medical practice and led to better understanding of normal structure and disease, safer treatment and better survival and outcomes for patients. This has only been possible because of the ceaseless innovation and deep collaboration between physics, engineering, computer science, radiologists and nuclear physicians. Technical innovations without clinical application have limited medical value, and constant feedback and development by clinicians of imaging techniques (also called "applications") for particular clinical indications has enabled medical imaging to become the indispensable clinical tool it is today.

Each imaging modality uses different forms of energy to create images. Most use electromagnetic radiation (EMR), from ionizing radiation (x-ray, fluoroscopy, angiography, CT and nuclear imaging), to non-ionizing radio waves (MRI), and even visible light (near-infrared or optical imaging). Uniquely, ultrasound does not use electromagnetic radiation but rather the pressure wave of high frequency sound to create its images. In each case, the interaction of energy with the body's tissues is captured, recorded, decoded and stored in order to create images that can be interpreted by medical practitioners. Each advance in medical imaging has in turn revealed more characteristics of specific diseases or anatomic structural changes in body tissues, has shown the anatomic effects of diseases and the responses to their surgical, medical or other treatment, and has led to a better understanding of how disease processes occur, evolve and resolve in response to various treatments.

Each imaging modality, because of the different interactions between the physical energy used and the different anatomic structures, as well as the mechanical design and technical constraints of each of the imaging systems, produces quite different kinds of images of various tissues, each of which is a partial representation of the imaged body part's structure and function. Imaging specialists have learned empirically – initially by trial and error and some accidental discovery, mostly by retrospective comparative analysis, and increasingly through prospective research – which imaging tests show various anatomic structures to best advantage, and which can reveal specific pathologies most accurately. It is a reality that no single imaging test can show all pathologies and all anatomic structures optimally (else this chapter would have little reason to be written), and that no imaging test can see all diseases in all parts of the body. Because there are now so many choices of medical imaging tests, the imaging specialist must have a concept of what the probable diagnoses are, in order to select the investigations most likely to provide the answer in that situation. Sometimes this task is straightforward (e. g., CT scan of the brain for acute bleeding, chest x-ray for pneumonia, or ultrasound for gall bladder stones), but often this decision is complex, and the best test cannot always be predicted *a priori*.

Because of this complexity, modern medical imaging tends to be multimodality, complementary and integrated – the radiologist must synthesise the clinical history, prior medical investigations, a broad and deep knowledge base, prior experience and often, more than one set of images of the same body part, perhaps using more than one imaging test, in order to develop a credible representation of normal anatomy and disease in that patient. In doing so, the radiologist is engaged in a practical epistemological task – trying to determine the "truth" for a particular patient by developing a hierarchical ranking of imaging information, in order to determine the reality of the disease state. In effect, the radiologist must decide whether and when to believe what he or she sees, and how to use the observations to come to a specific diagnosis. Such a state of belief arises from a combination of training, learning from the experience of others, learning from one's own experience, and correlation with the relevant clinical features and any subsequent histopathology or surgical pathology, which remains in many (but not all) instances the "gold standard" by which imaging truth is judged.

Medical image interpretation appears simple in many cases, and some expert practitioners can make it appear even simpler; however, it has many recognised pitfalls:

–   Images often contain technique-specific artefacts that may be confused with disease
–   Normal anatomic variants may mimic disease
–   Some diseases may be mistaken for normal structures or normal variants
–   Some diseases cannot be diagnosed with specific imaging techniques
–   Some diseases are only well-seen using special techniques or from specific anatomic viewpoints
–   Many diseases have similar and/or overlapping appearances
–   Important imaging findings may not be perceived by the reader
–   Important imaging findings may be perceived but dismissed erroneously as unimportant
–   Important imaging findings may be very subtle or interpretable only if the radiologist suspects a specific condition

Thus in more complex cases, a deep knowledge of conditions that may affect certain organs in concert, acute observational skills and deductive reasoning are needed for accurate diagnosis. Often, radiologists are unable to explain exactly how they came to a specific (correct) diagnosis. Sometimes, "gut instinct" and intuition are cited, but the process is a complex, partly conscious and partly subconscious one that is ingrained through years of training, observation of thousands of examples over many years, and the ability to integrate, correlate and associate knowledge across different fields of medicine and parts of the body. In this way a radiologist can often correctly deduce a specific diagnosis, even if he or she has never seen an example of this condition before! This process of imaging-based diagnostics has largely defied scientific attempts to analyse and break down how its results are achieved, except in the simplest cases.

Imaging has permeated its way into all aspects of medicine, and whether practitioners call themselves medical imagers or not, most use medical imaging as an integral part of their routine practice – either as requesters and users of medical imaging investigations and procedures, or as practitioners for whom some form of imaging is inseparable from their practice. There are many groups who are not usually thought of as imaging specialists, but who often perform imaging within their own departments or clinic facilities, including:

– Anesthetists
– Cardiologists
– Ophthalmologists
– Gastroenterologists
– Obstetricians and gynecologists
– Orthopaedic surgeons
– Pain management specialists
– Radiation oncologists
– Renal physicians
– Urologists
– Vascular surgeons

In general, most of these practitioners confine their imaging practice to one or two types of imaging tests, and only a very few are dedicated imaging specialists in their own narrow field, conducting imaging requests on referral from other practitioners, and practising little or no clinical medicine. These specialists in many ways share more in common with radiologists and nuclear physicians than their original craft group. The complexity of modern imaging demands that the imaging practitioner is dedicated to the task of imaging diagnosis in order to be truly expert. While there are those who claim that knowing a specific test for a specific organ enables them to be as expert in that field, inevitably they fail to appreciate the entire range of pathologies that may present themselves in what is increasingly a totally 3-dimensional presentation of all that is normal and abnormal in the imaged part of the body. For example, it has been shown that reading coronary artery CT scans without complete review of the full chest will miss, overlook or ignore significant pathology in the remainder of the imaged chest in 16% of cases (Johnson 2010).

Perhaps unfortunately, the very rapidity and apparent simplicity by which most imaging tests can be performed today, the seductively high quality of modern imaging, and the ease and clarity with which some diagnoses can be depicted, has led many to believe that medical imaging interpretation of the highest standard is available to all without any special (or perhaps very limited) training. This is an intellectual trap, and belies the extensive training and expertise, broad and deep knowledge base, understanding of imaging technology, analytic skills, the myriad appearances in different imaging contexts of various diseases and the ability to communicate such findings precisely and effectively in writing that are acquired by the expert radiologist. It is a also a truism that only radiologists are routinely highly trained and expert in all aspects of cross-sectional, 3D and multiplanar anatomy of virtually all parts of the body. It is clear that clarification and better understanding of the nature and complexity of radiological expertise would be of benefit in resisting attempts to trivialise the depth and complexity of multimodality medical imaging interpretation and diagnosis.

This chapter will briefly enumerate the different types of medical imaging available today, explain how such imaging methods each inform different aspects of understanding of the complexities of the human body, and discuss some philosophical aspects of the work of the medical imaging specialist. First, I will explain the nature of commonly available imaging tests, and explain how they work and how they differ. Next, I will discuss how medical imaging is now effectively entirely virtual and realised only on computers, with the medical image today having only an indirect relationship to the reality that it depicts. I will explain how medical imaging has influenced our ability to diagnose, treat and monitor the patient much more accurately than in its absence, and how this has in turn greatly increased our understanding of disease and anatomy. I will expound on the nature of radiological expertise and how radiologists construct a conception of imaging "truth" for any specific examination or patient. Finally, I will close with a brief discussion on the value of a philosophical grounding in medical imaging.

X-RAY BASED IMAGING

X-rays are the simplest form of medical imaging. X-rays are a form of electromagnetic radiation composed of moderately high energy photons that can pass through solid objects such as the human body, and when captured by a detector on the other side of the body, can create images. Although in theoretical terms x-rays are no different to low energy cosmic rays or gamma radiation emitted by many radioisotopes, in practice they differ enormously. X-rays are generated as a high intensity beam of photons by a device called an x-ray tube using a very high electrical voltage that can be instantaneously be turned on and off. The beam can be accurately directed, modified in energy and filtered to suit the tissue of interest, can be instantaneous or continuous in output, and is readily controlled with the touch of a few buttons or even automatically. This differs substantially from radioisotopes and other natural sources of electromagnetic radiation, that are generally of much lower intensity, are constantly emitting radiation, have no directionality, and cannot be easily adjusted or directed.

Medical X-rays are absorbed variably by different tissues (e. g., air, calcium fat, bone, water) so that they appear different on the captured image. The original detector used by Röntgen in 1895 was a sheet of photographic film in a light-tight envelope, and film was the mainstay of radiographic image capture and storage until very recently. Film has the virtue of simplicity and low per image cost, but also has very low radiation sensitivity when used alone for x-ray capture – the silver halide emulsion captures only a tiny fraction of the x-rays that pass through it (after all, x-rays, as has been already stated, pass through solid matter easily). Technical advances in the mid-20th century replaced direct capture by film with fluorescent screens of increasing efficiency that exposed film with visible light, and finally digital detectors of initially indirect and more recently direct x-ray photon conversion design, leading to much lower radiation doses and improved image quality over time. This process has taken almost a century, so that modern radiologists have no experience of the limitations of these older systems. Recently, a 115-year old first generation x-ray system was resurrected for testing and producing medical x-rays (of phantoms). This system's radiation output was measured, and required 1,500 times the dose of a modern x-ray system to produce a readable, but rather low quality x-ray image (Kemerink 2011)!

Fluoroscopy is the real-time display of x-ray images, originally using a thin coating of fluorescent compounds such as barium platinocyanide on a sheet of glass that was held over the patient on the opposite side of the x-ray beam. This effect of x-rays on such fluorescent compounds was discovered by Röntgen, and was instrumental in his discovery of x-rays. Fluoroscopy was ground-breaking because of its ability to depict motion in real-time (unlike x-rays, which produced instantaneous snapshot images). For decades however, the very weak light emission of such fluorescent materials made imaging difficult, requiring thorough dark adaptation of the visual system (which takes about 30 minutes) in order to adequately see the faint images produced. Until the mid-1970's, radiologists performing fluoroscopy would routinely wear red goggles even in normal lighting (sometimes even on the way to work!) to develop and preserve this dark adaptation in between cases. Fluoroscopy was made much more practical with the application of television and video technologies from the 1970's onwards, to enable bright, clear images to be shown on a cathode ray screen in normal room lighting. Fluoroscopy often requires the introduction of radio-opaque substances into the body to depict different organs such as the stomach or intestine. Insoluble barium sulfate suspensions or soluble iodine-based agents are used to outline the hollow gastrointestinal tract or other body cavities. When iodine-based compounds are injected directly into the blood vessels to show their flow and anatomy, this is termed angiography.

X-rays, fluoroscopy and angiography depict flattened images of the entire thickness of the body part projected onto a single plane. Such planar imaging methods simplify the 3-dimensional (3D) appearance of the organ or tissue and permit a global overview of an entire body part or even the whole body in a single image. Conversely, they also make it difficult to differentiate some structures that overlap, or to determine the precise localisation of most structures without additional projections from different angles. To overcome such limitations of anatomic localisation, various forms of tomography (or slice imaging, from the Greek *tomos*, a cut or section) were developed. To perform tomography with x-rays, mechanically complex machines that moved the x-ray tube in one direction and the film in the opposite direction were invented in order to blur structures out of the plane of effective focus, leaving the plane of interest in focus. However, such images were affected by an intrinsic and unavoidable lack of sharpness, low image contrast, and lack of sensitivity to soft tissue structures. They were primarily of value in imaging bony diseases or conditions where exogenous contrast agents had been introduced into the body but contrast was too low to see the full details using conventional planar x-rays.

Computed tomography (CT) also uses x-rays as an energy source, but the x-ray tube is not static; it rotates around the patient at high speed using a highly focussed beam, with an array of x-ray detectors mechanically linked on the opposite side of the patient. The detectors collect the x-rays passing through the patient, differentiating the variable absorption of x-rays at different points around the body, and feed the information to a powerful computer, which in turn reconstructs slice-by-slice images of the imaged body part. Such images eliminated the unsharp images of x-ray tomography, and enabled for the first time direct slice-based imaging *across* the long axis of the body (conventional tomography was limited to the long axis for physical and mechanical reasons), and became the first imaging tool that could see both soft tissues and bone almost equally well.

Curiously, the invention of CT was made possible by the success of the pop group The Beatles, whose enormous revenues allowed their recording company EMI to fund the research of one of their employees, the engineer Godfrey Houns-field (Rossoff 2008), whose work in inventing the CT scanner was rewarded with the Nobel Prize in Medicine in 1979. The fundamental principles of back projection reconstruction that enabled CT image reconstruction to be performed rapidly had been published many years earlier. The full history of the development of CT is beyond the scope of this chapter, but the reader is referred to the work of Filler (Filler 2009) for more detail.

Using CT, for the first time 3-dimensional anatomy and diseases such as bleeding, stroke and tumours could be imaged directly, not merely by inferring their presence through displacements or deformation of normal structures. CT has continued to develop and is now capable of imaging the whole body in a few seconds, and even the beating heart in exquisite anatomic detail.

NON-X-RAY IMAGING

X-rays were used for imaging the body from the very beginning; the very first x-ray image recorded was that of the bones of Röntgen's wife's hand. All subsequent x-ray imaging from fluoroscopy to angiography to CT scan, digital radiography and mammography has depended on refining the application of the same energy source and its accompanying imaging technologies. In parallel with these huge technological advances, physicists and engineers realised that other sources of energy could be applied to perform medical imaging. Thus imaging techniques that do not use x-rays were adapted from other technologies in order to produce medical images. Ultrasound (US) was developed from sonar technologies used for submarine detection in World War II, magnetic resonance imaging (MRI) arose from the chemical analysis method called nuclear magnetic resonance (NMR), radioisotope imaging or nuclear medicine (NM) was developed to spatially map the distribution of administered radioisotopes (and thus borrowed heavily from the development of fluoroscopy before it). More recently, optical imaging using near infrared (NIR) light has been developed in a variety of forms, both planar and cross-sectional; this work has relied heavily on work by Britton Chance and his colleagues since the 1950's that differential absorption of such light could differentiate, quantitate and even visualise various metabolic processes *in vitro* and *in vivo* (Chance 1952, Mancini 1994, Yodh & Chance 1995). Optical and other alternative forms of imaging including thermography, electrical impedance mapping and microwave imaging have yet to achieve any practical clinical use or widespread application however, so will not be further discussed.

Ultrasound

The term "ultrasound" applies to sound waves with a frequency above the audible range of human hearing (greater than 20,000 cycles per second, or Hertz [Hz]). Ultrasound was discovered and researched intensively in the 19th century. No less a scientist than Lord Rayleigh, who received the Nobel Prize in Physics in 1904 for his discovery of argon, is credited with virtually single-handedly founding the science of ultrasound with his two volume treatise, "The Theory of Sound" published in 1877 (Nobelprize.org, 2011).

The piezoelectric effect, where a solid material creates an electrical charge in response to pressure, and can conversely convert an electrical charge to a pressure change, was first reported by the Curie brothers in 1880. This phenomenon is essential for the construction of ultrasound transducers. Ultrasound owes much to the earlier development of SONAR for the detection of underwater submarines using the "hydrophone" instrument by Chilowsky and Langevin in 1915 (Newman 1998). Despite various attempts to use ultrasound in humans before and after World War II, it was Douglass Howry and W. Roderick Bliss who developed the first clinically usable B-mode ultrasound scanner in 1949, and the first linear water bath scanner in 1951. In 1961, W. Wright and E. Myers developed the linear contact scanner (Newman 1998).

Ultrasound was the first intrinsically tomographic imaging method. Initially bistable (i. e., images were only black or white, showing mainly bony structures), ultrasound was first applied to imaging the body experimentally in the late 1940's, and entered clinical use in obstetrics about 10 years later through the pioneering efforts of Ian Donald, an obstetrician from Glasgow, who with a fellow obstetrician John Macvicar and the engineer Tom Brown, developed the first contact compound scanner. This led to the first report of clinical ultrasound in The Lancet (Donald 1958). The B-mode contact compound scanner was progressively refined but remained difficult to use and required extensive training and hand-eye coordination to produce reasonable quality images.

A series of subsequent technical developments made ultrasound dramatically easier to use and more intuitive to learn; these included the development of grey-scale ultrasound by George Kossoff and colleagues in Australia (Kossoff et al, 1973) and real-time ultrasound, invented by Walter Krause and Richard Soldner in 1965 (Woo 2002). Until the mid-1980's, it was not clear whether hand-held real-time contact ultrasound would be superior to multi-transducer water-bath ultrasound. Subsequently, very rapid commercial development of hand-held transducers and dramatic improvements in image quality led to real-time ultrasound replacing all other forms of ultrasound in routine diagnostic practice.

Medical ultrasound today is performed using a narrow beam of high frequency sound that is propagated into a body part and reflected from different tissue interfaces. The image is reconstructed from the reflected sound waves received by the ultrasound probe. However, ultrasound is blocked by bone and gas, and is typically unable to produce good quality images of a large volume of tissue. This physical limitations of ultrasound means it cannot be used to depict the entire body. Nevertheless, its lack of ionizing radiation and exquisite soft tissue detail (in the absence of gas or bone) make it indispensable in many medical applications, particularly in evaluation of pregnancy, the liver, kidneys and the musculoskeletal system. The development of miniaturised endocavitary and endoluminal ultrasound probes has meant that high resolution ultrasound of previously occult body parts such as the pancreas, the prostate gland and even the inner surface of blood vessels can be routinely obtained.

MRI

MRI was developed from NMR, a powerful chemical analysis tool that is still in use today. Although Paul Lauterbur was the first to create a tomographic MRI image based on the filtered back projection method that Hounsfield had used for CT scanning (Lauterbur 1973), it was Raymond Damadian who conceived of a machine capable of scanning the human body using NMR (Damadian 1974), to detect cancer using a technique he had reported earlier (Damadian 1971). Rapid development of MRI technologies and methods occurred during the early 1980's, and the first clinical systems entered clinical practice in 1983, some 50 years after the principle of NMR related chemical shift was discovered independently by Bloch and Purcell. A full account of the development of MRI was recently published by Filler (Filler 2009).

MRI creates images of the body by placing the patient into a powerful magnetic field, and essentially turning the patient into a weak radio transmitter, emitting encoded, highly tuned radio waves that can be received by a set of antennae, and decoded by a computer into cross-sectional images. It produces images of heretofore unprecedented quality, and depicts anatomy and diseases that could not be seen otherwise. An explosion of medical knowledge followed the introduction of MRI as its unique flexibility and sensitivity was exploited to display and explain diseases that had been previously poorly understood. The ability to detect and measure chemical metabolites is the strength of NMR as a scientific tool, and it is now possible to use MR spectroscopic imaging to map of tissue concentrations of different chemical species such as citrate and sodium *in vivo* noninvasively. The discovery of the blood oxygen level dependent (BOLD) effect (Ogawa et al., 1990), which reveals different signals from blood with normal and reduced oxygen levels, enabled MRI to detect and map the function of brain regionally in a flexible and repeatable manner that was not possible with other methods. This technique of functional MRI (fMRI) has led in turn to a revolution in understanding how the human brain works, transforming our understanding of not only the brain's mechanistic functions but also providing some insights into where more abstract abilities such as ideation, language and learning are located and how these functions may interact. MRI is also able to determine how tissues are organised, and to depict this organisation using diffusion-weighted imaging (DWI), which when processed to extract directional information, is called diffusion tensor imaging (DTI), which in its most startling form shows the connections between parts of the brain with other parts. Thus in a single examination, MRI can depict anatomic structure, intrinsic connectivity, blood flow and chemical composition.

Nuclear Medicine

Practical high quality radioisotope imaging was enabled by the invention of the planar multi-detector gamma camera in the 1950's by Hal O. Anger (Anger 1953). Prior to this, the spatial localisation of radioactivity in the human body was recorded using devices called rectilinear scanners, which were strip-based radiation detectors that moved continuously from the patient's head downwards, and which recorded their counts as marks on a strip or sheet of paper or film. The development of the gamma camera enabled the photons emitted from radioisotopes to be imaged fairly rapidly with high sensitivity. The development of different physiologic tracer molecules that could be readily labelled with widely available isotopes such as technetium-99m permitted imaging of a wide variety of physiologic processes to be visualised over time, such as the excretion of bile, the emptying of the stomach, the leakage of blood and the deposition of bone. Gamma imaging was initially planar, but by borrowing methods used in CT, slice-based gamma imaging is now possible.

More recently cellular metabolism such as the usage of glucose can be assessed with positron emission tomography (PET) using a radioactive analog of glucose (18-fluorodeoxyglucose, 18-FDG), the development of which was crucial to the current success of this imaging method (Do 1978). Positrons are positively charged electrons that are emitted by a small number of unstable radioisotopes. These particles, when they encounter electrons in any substance, self-destruct and create two photons of a fixed high energy that radiate away from the destruction point at 180° to each other. Instead of a plate of scintillation detectors, as is found in a planar gamma camera, the PET scanner has a ring of detectors around the patient; this design evolved from an initially single plane PET camera to a circular multidetector array through the work of Robertson *et al* (Robertson 1973) and Cho *et al* (Cho 1975). Rapid computational analysis of events detected simultaneously on opposite sides of the ring permits the PET scanner can reconstruct a map of the location of positron-electron interactions in the body, with greater precision and better signal-to-noise than traditional gamma imaging permits. However, it was not until the development of the combined or hybrid PET-CT scanner by Townsend and Nutt in the late 1990's that it became practical to accurately and routinely localise abnormal activity detected by the PET imaging system; this in turn led to rapid growth in utilisation and widespread dissemination of PET/CT systems around the world.

IONISING RADIATION AND HARM

X-rays and radioactivity can damage body tissues by a process called ionization. Ionization occurs when photons are sufficiently energetic so as to change the electrical charge of molecules they interact with. Ionization can thus damage the fundamental genetic molecule deoxyribonucleic acid (DNA) in cells, and so cause genetic defects, cell death or even cancer. Sometimes this effect is used deliberately to treat diseases by destroying tissues (e. g., radiotherapy).

In medical imaging with x-rays and radioisotopes, the imaging expert has to balance the prospect of delivering harmful radiation whilst gathering potentially life-saving information about the patient. This introduces an ethical aspect to such medical practice that may not be as critical if the imaging method (such as ultrasound or MRI) was thought to be mostly harmless. There is widespread lack of understanding by the medical and general community about the levels of radiation involved in different imaging tests. Sometimes there is an over-reaction, with excessive concern about relatively trivial or nonsignificant levels of radiation exposure (e. g., whole body airport scanners, fear of thyroid radiation from mammography), yet a similar lack of appreciation of the very real levels of radiation dose delivered by some interventional radiology procedures or CT scans, which have been documented to cause at least hair loss and radiation skin burns.

CT scan is currently the highest source of radiation exposure to the general public. The indiscriminate use of CT scan has, on occasion, led to excessive radiation doses to individuals, particularly using multiphase multislice spiral CT. Interventional radiology procedures often use fluoroscopy, and long complex procedures may lead to relatively large patient exposures that exceed even those of CT in a focal area of the body. This is particularly true if the patient requires repeated interventions over a short period of time. Such radiation exposure also carries an increased lifelong risk for adverse effects such as genetic defects or even cancer. This effect is more pronounced in children and young adults.

There is thus an ethical principle in medical imaging to ensure that the lowest doses feasible are used for any imaging test that uses ionising radiation. This principle is known by the acronym ALARA (As Low As Reasonably Achievable). Since repeated surveys have shown that the majority of nonradiologist clinicians have minimal, limited or even misleading knowledge of the typical doses delivered by diagnostic and interventional procedures, the radiologist has an important "gatekeeper" role in trying to keep individual and community radiation exposure to a reasonable minimum. Conversely, clinical practitioners who have come to rely more and more on the detection or exclusion of significant disease through imaging want unfettered and essentially unlimited access to imaging in order to aid their clinical decision-making; such clinicians generally resent any attempts to reduce their access to imaging, or for radiologists to resist a request for imaging that the radiologist considers inappropriate. More recently there has been a push to recognise the rights of the patient in the decision to perform imaging tests where x-rays or other forms of ionising radiation may be utilised; however, for now this remains logistically challenging and has not reached a level where conceptual acceptance is widespread in the medical community.

The whole "life-cycle" of the medical imaging investigation process has many potential pitfalls and points of weakness where harm to the patient may occur. Miscommunication or omission of relevant clinical information by the referring clinician, failure to adequately inform patients of specific relevant risks, incorrect tests or tests of the wrong body part, missed abnormalities or misinterpretation of imaging findings by the radiologist, and failures in communication of the final report to the clinician in a timely fashion, are far more likely to cause harm to the patient than the imaging test itself. The radiologist has then an ethical duty of care to ensure that the entire imaging cycle, from the initiating request for an imaging test to the communication of the final result to the referring physician, is appropriate and of suitable quality, in order to ensure that optimal outcomes ensue.

VIRTUALISATION AND ABSTRACTION OF MEDICAL IMAGES

At the beginning of medical imaging, the image detector and storage device was the same, i.e., a sheet of photographic film. In the quest for reductions in dose, increased quality and facility of display, direct film capture of x-rays was improved using fluorescent screens, then digital capture of fluorescent screens or phosphors, and more recently, direct capture using purely digital technologies. The modern medical image is exclusively captured, processed and displayed using computers, is entirely virtual, and has lost its original direct physical connection between the energy source and the image embodied by an x-ray photon striking a sheet of photographic film. Film has become simply one of many ways to display the final image, and while easily viewed and highly portable, lacks the power and flexibility of digital display.

At the same time, the computerised capture, display and storage of images means images can be transmitted, reprocessed and reanalysed both qualitatively and quantitatively in ways that were previously impractical, if not impossible. Thus it is possible for a series of images acquired under very specific circumstances to be interpreted and analysed by another team of people far away, both temporally and spatially. This can be a boon, when expert opinion can be sought remotely, or a failing if the specific context and techniques of that study are incorrectly integrated into the diagnostic process.

This virtualisation of medical imaging has occurred across all imaging modalities today, which has profound implications for the perception of tissue structure, function and diseases by medical experts reading such images. The danger inherent in this virtualisation and the startlingly high quality of modern images is that we tend to believe them without questioning their accuracy, representation and veracity. Most medical practitioners do not realise that many medical images carry some form of intrinsic spatial or temporal distortions and artifacts, and that such distortions or artifacts may be difficult to perceive or may even be misleading. Although uncommon and unlikely, it is possible to artificially create disease, diagnose one disease as another, over-represent the importance of imaging findings in disease, or obscure true disease with any imaging test, and the understanding of this potential is hard-won by medical imaging specialists through rigorous training, self-learning and experience.

An unintended consequence of the drive to develop better, faster and higher resolution imaging has been the proliferation of data that this generates. In the past, imaging of the chest mean perhaps 2–3 separate x-ray exposures and 2–3 films to interpret. A CT scan of the chest in 1990 produced about 20–30 slices. Today, a CT of the chest may produce several hundred images. Scanning of the entire body, which used to take more than an hour, can now be acquired in under 1 minute. Such speed has created a new problem for radiologists in particular – that of gigantic datasets that have to be reviewed, interpreted, reconstructed, displayed and analysed in a manner that stretches the abilities of the human visual processing system (Andriole 2011). This problem is not confined to CT, of course – MRI and nuclear imaging, especially PET/CT, may also create enormous imaging datasets that require new methods of storage, processing, analysis and interpretation.

Ultimately all medical images are abstract representations of reality, and require a degree of abstract ideation within a conceptual representational framework in order to relate an image to a part of the patient that is otherwise invisible to the naked eye. Radiologists, through extensive training and experience, become very good at this visual abstraction task, to the point where they rarely have to think about it. Various studies have shown that expert radiologist can identify an abnormality in one or more medical images within a few seconds, often immediately. When asked to draw an abnormality, the radiologist will draw the lesion and place it in its broader anatomic context; a lay or nonexpert person sees the pathology only as a fragment within a complex sea of findings, and is unable to determine the significance of the key abnormality.

IMPACT OF BETTER VISUALISATION ON MEDICINE

"A picture is worth a thousand words"
– *Anonymous*

It is difficult to underestimate the impact that medical imaging has had on medical practice. The effect has been transformational, with a large majority of common diseases now readily visible on various forms of imaging. Where previously clinical judgement, deduction, inference and supposition was used to determine whether a patient had a disease such as an abscess or a tumour, today that disease can be depicted, its size and precise location determined, and the degree of involvement of local structures, or associated findings remote from the disease can be easily obtained through imaging.

Until the advent of the CT scanner, in most large hospitals the commonest operation was the exploratory laparotomy, where the surgeon would open the abdominal cavity to see what might be happening in a patient. Today, such surgery is much less common wherever CT scans are routinely used to interrogate the abdomen and pelvis. Surgeons now depend heavily on CT scans to provide them with a road map for the operation. Imaging remains imperfect and insensitive to small amounts of disease, so it is not uncommon for surgeons to find additional pathology at the time of operation that was not diagnosed beforehand. Nevertheless, modern imaging has dramatically improved surgical planning. Most recently, surgeons have started to install imaging devices and displays in the operating suite, to permit more accurate planning and guidance during the operation.

In a similar vein, radiotherapy planning was, until about 15 years ago, entirely dependent on planar x-rays. X-rays are by nature poor at depicting soft tissue diseases such as cancer, which meant that radiotherapists had to estimate where the disease was likely to be, and treat an area much larger than the estimated disease size to ensure the disease was fully encompassed by the treatment beam. For tissues that do not move much, this was satisfactory. However, it was impossible to conform to curved objects, and movements during treatment were difficult to compensate for. Radiation injury to adjacent normal tissues was the norm. The integration of CT scans and more recently MRI scans into radiotherapy treatment planning, together with 3D conformal radiotherapy (where the radiation dose can be focussed tightly using computer control onto a 3D volume visible on CT or MRI to maximise local dose and minimise adjacent tissue damage), has made it possible to treat disease in a much more accurate fashion than in the past.

Interventional radiology is a discipline within Radiology that arose from angiography. Abnormalities in blood vessels can be treated using angiography to guide the patient's treatment in real-time, yet another form of image-guided therapy. Narrowed arteries can be widened, bleeding arteries can be blocked, swellings in arteries that rupture (called aneurysms) can be occluded, and abnormal connections between arteries and veins (called arteriovenous malformations or arteriovenous fistulae) can be blocked and disconnected without the need for surgery. The advent of cross-sectional imaging of the body with ultrasound, then CT and MRI, mean that an abnormal fluid collection (e. g., an abscess or blocked kidney) could be located and drained using small needles and tubes instead of open surgery, and that tissues suspicious for cancer or infection could be sampled very precisely and safely under imaging guidance, again without the need for surgery. These advances have led to safer, faster, cheaper and more effective treatments in many cases than traditional surgical methods – so much so that in modern hospitals most patients with an infected collection of fluid are managed by radiologically guided drainage rather than surgery.

More recently, the development of various therapeutic devices that can destroy cancers by the arterial route or by placement of treatment probes to treat a tumour has created the field of interventional oncology. Cancers may be injected with bone cement (cementoplasty), frozen (cryotherapy), heated and coagulated (laser, radiofrequency or microwave ablation), shocked by a controlled electrical current (electroporation), directly infused with chemotherapy (intra-arterial chemoinfusion), have their blood supply occluded alone (embolisation) or in combination with chemotherapy infusion (chemoembolisation), or treated by implantation of highly radioactive beads (radioembolisation). These treatments are performed by a variety of different medical specialists, most often interventional radiologists, and always under some form of imaging guidance. For all of these interventional treatments, the patient usually recovers very quickly with far fewer side effects and complications than with traditional surgery. None of this would be possible without real-time imaging during the procedure.

For many nonsurgical disciplines, imaging is crucial because it permits nonsurgical treatment efficacy to be monitored. The response of cancers to chemotherapy cannot be accurately determined with CT and MRI scans. The reduction in extent of pneumonia in response to antibiotics requires at least repeated chest x-rays. The healing of a fracture is best shown on x-rays, and the spread of cancer to the bones is best demonstrated on nuclear isotope bone scans. From general practitioners to internal medicine physicians, the ability of imaging to accurately demonstrate the effects of their treatments is not only useful for their own satisfaction but also can guide treatment changes if the disease is not responding.

A consequence of all this evolution of treatment guided by high quality, readily available imaging is that treatments have become more sophisticated, more precise, more effective and with fewer side-effects and complications for the patient. Imaging can be clearly said to have improved patient care and outcomes.

UNDERSTANDING OF PATHOPHYSIOLOGY

An aspect of improved medical imaging over the last 50 years that is perhaps under-recognised is the way it has informed and transformed our understanding of disease processes. Processes that previously could only be observed in a longitudinal fashion in the most crude manner, or indirectly, were suddenly revealed to have a completely different, or much more subtle and variable nature in time and space than originally suspected. An example of this is the progressive nature of normal and disordered myelination of the infant and child brain, something which could not be properly assessed prior to the advent of MRI.

Some mysterious aspects of patient symptomatology, signs or even biochemical changes were clarified by imaging of the anatomic status of a particular pathology. An example of this is the nature of pituitary dwarfism, which can have traumatic, developmental, toxic, inflammatory and neoplastic causes. The application of MRI to the study of this condition enabled for the first time revelation that some forms of dwarfism were due to a failure of the normal development of the pituitary stalk, something that was not previously suspected (Kelly 1988).

Even now in the genomic era, medical imaging continues to be of great value as the phenotypic expression of genetic differences between variants of a particular disease may be obvious on imaging, which is still cheaper and faster than individual genotyping. For example, some types of hereditary muscular dystrophy can differ greatly in the MRI appearance of specific muscles (Mercuri 2005).

Phenotypical changes due to alterations in physiology that are elucidated through angiogenesis imaging, perfusion imaging and metabolic imaging are not suited to genomic testing and bear little relation to the here and now of the type of response of a disease to treatment. This is now routinely applied in clinical practice, with 18-FDG-PET able to much more sensitively detect early spread and metabolic response to cancer therapy than CT or MRI in tumours (and much, much more accurately than any clinical assessment) such as gastrointestinal stromal tumours, lymphoma and metastatic colorectal carcinoma.

The advent of CT scan and ultrasound (US) revealed much that x-ray had been unable to clarify except through indirect deduction and inference. Haemorrhage into the brain became directly visible, and could be graded and quantified and localised; prior to these technologies, pneumoencephalography, ventriculography and angiography were used to infer the presence of severe mass effects; they could not directly show the haemorrhage. With CT and US for the first time, soft tissues could be interrogated with great detail and accuracy without using exogenous contrast agents in a natively tomographic (i. e., slice-based) fashion; projectional x-ray methods had been developed to image slices of tissue but because of intrinsically low image contrast, these were not suited to imaging of soft tissues except for perhaps the lungs. With increasing sophistication, CT and US have completely replaced plain x-ray tomography. Interestingly, despite having been in widespread use for more than 30 years, CT and US continue to be developed towards better and better image quality, and now permit routine depiction of pathologies that had previously been poorly visualised or only inferred even with the same technologies. For example, the direct depiction of the size, extent and severity a tear within a tendon is now commonplace and exquisitely shown on modern ultrasound systems, whereas this could only be imagined and inferred when US was initially used for this purpose. Even today we are still learning new features of normal and disease depicted by the progressive advances in these imaging technologies.

The extraordinary image quality of MRI enabled even greater levels of sophistication in image analysis than was possible with CT or US. Where both these techniques rely largely on a single tissue tissue characteristic to create image contrast and differentiate between tissues (electron density or attenuation for CT, and echogenicity or acoustic impedance for US), MRI is almost infinitely flexible in its ability to literally tune in and tune out signal from different tissues at different times – the main limitations to its flexibility are the imagination of those designing the complex radiofrequency pulse sequences that elucidate such differences, the design and construction of the hardware to receive the signals with high fidelity, and the software required to decode these signals, reconstruct the images and display them in a clinically meaningful way.

MRI thus, unlike any imaging modality before or since, is able to depict the same tissue in many different ways, with the signal differences between tissues depending on many factors, including:

–   Chemical composition
–   Cellularity
–   Intrinsic structural organisation
–   Water content
–   Perfusion
–   Bulk tissue motion
–   Blood flow and oxygen usage

- Microscopic diffusion of water
- Microscopic variations in magnetic field within tissues

Even early on, it became clear that MRI was showing information that did not have an obvious gross anatomic correlation and required further systematic investigation. Why, for example, was the posterior pituitary gland brighter than the anterior on certain imaging sequences? And why did this signal equalise in some patients with diabetes mellitus (a condition that causes abnormally high urinary output because of the lack of the hormone vasopressin, which is secreted by the posterior pituitary) but not in others? Why did haemorrhage, which on CT when fresh appeared bright, and gradually faded progressively with age, have such highly variable signal intensities at different times of its evolution? Why did malformations of the corpus callosum, a developmental disorder of the major interhemispheric white matter bundle between the left and right cerebral hemispheres, progress in severity from the back to the front? Why was the bone marrow on T1-weighted imaging bright in most patients, grey in others and dark in a small proportion?

The quest for answers to many of these questions over the last 25 years of clinical MRI has led us to understand the organisation of tissues better, the structure and development of organs more completely, the biochemistry of some processes better (e. g., the progressive chemical changes in the degradation of a blood clot), the physiology of disease processes more thoroughly (e. g., the alteration in perfusion and capillary permeability of cancers in response to chemotherapy) and the molecular basis for the tissue signal changes we were seeing. In the process our understanding of many diseases has greatly increased, and has transformed practice.

The use of MR diffusion and perfusion imaging of stroke has led to much greater understanding of this once fairly mysterious disorder, and has directly led to new methods to try to minimise or even actively reverse the impact of such events. And this understanding has enabled us to translate the science and knowledge so gained back to modern multislice CT perfusion imaging, which is more logistically feasible in the acute stroke patient. This is an excellent example of the ability to image in a sophisticated manner transforming the clinical understanding of disease, leading to new concepts in disease management and treatment, and in a positive feedback fashion, leading to new methods of imaging to make such treatments faster and more effective for more patients.

Radioisotope imaging has always relied on specific pathophysiologic effects to depict normal and diseased tissues. Nuclear imaging includes gamma-ray projectional imaging (rather analogous to x-rays), single photon computed tomography (SPECT, analogous to CT) and positron emission tomography (PET, which has no real analogue in radiology). It relies on the ability of a specific molecular species which has been tagged with a radioactive tracer such as 99m-Technetium, 131-Iodine, or 18-Fluorine, to be distributed either actively or passively by a specific tissue (e. g., the renal tubule, the myocardium) or a specific metabolic process (e. g., new bone deposition, or utilisation of glucose). Nuclear imaging is intrinsically far more sensitive to diseases that take up such tracers than any radiologic imaging process, including MRI. However, if the disease is highly specific for the tracer, then anatomic localisation of what may be a single small hot spot in the body becomes highly problematic – for this reason, hybrid imaging instruments such as the PET/CT scanner, have been developed to facilitate accurate localisation of such findings in 3D space. With sophisticated tracer design, it is possible to image many processes *in vivo* in addition to those possible through radiological methods; some of these include:

–   Tissue use of glucose in the heart, brain, cancers and infection
–   Low tissue oxygen levels in cancer
–   Plaque deposition in the brain in Alzheimer Disease
–   Metabolic activity of the heart muscles
–   Function of the thyroid gland

It can be seen then that imaging today is not just about depiction of what is present in the body. It is about revealing both structure and function of different components of specific organs, and through this revelation, leading to better understanding of the organ and the perturbations that occur in health and disease. Through such imaging we have been able to devise new methods of treatment and monitoring of disease status, which in turn have driven the development of even more sophisticated imaging methods. This virtuous cycle is an intrinsic aspect of modern medical imaging, has become pervasively embedded into routine practice (though perhaps now to an unhealthy degree), and is happening so quickly that clinical practitioners are struggling to keep pace with the changes, and lay people are at risk of being increasingly confused and misinformed about the potential benefits and risks of imaging.

RADIOLOGISTS NEED PHILOSOPHY

Fundamentally, radiologists are observers and empiricists, and both infer and deduce diagnoses and clinical decision-making through observation in day to day practice with real patients. Much of radiological knowledge is based on systematic empirical gathering of observations by generations of preceding radiologists, and are often based on lists of diagnoses linked by their imaging findings known as *gamuts*. In most cases the individual items on such lists have almost nothing in common with each other except for the fact that they may produce an imaging finding that looks a lot like another disease. A typical example is the gamut for a hot spot in a bone found on nuclear medicine bone scanning:

–   Recent fracture due to trauma
–   Old fracture due to trauma
–   Infection of the bone (osteomyelitis)
–   Recent surgery at the site
–   Benign focal bone tumour (many types)

- Malignant focal bone tumour (many types)
- Cancer spread from another organ (many types)
- Overall bone weakness leading to bone failure (another type of fracture)

Another example is the gamut for bright spots in the white matter of the brain of a middle-aged person on T2-weighted MRI, which is an extremely common finding:

- Normal variant from widening of the fluid around tiny white matter blood vessels
- Old small stroke
- Recent small stroke
- Focal recent haemorrhage (blood clot)
- Developmental malformation of the blood vessels
- Multiple sclerosis plaque (demyelination)
- Other cause of demyelination
- Previous trauma
- Post-operative track or scar
- Infection (many types)
- Cancer spread from other organs (many types)

As one can immediately see, the subsequent investigation pathway and treatment for the patient would differ enormously depending on the diagnosis selected by the imaging specialist from these lists. In order for the specialist to decide which of these entities represents that particular patient's condition, it is crucial for that specialist to know what differentiates each of these entities – whether that be a specific combination of imaging features, the behaviour of the "lesion" with different imaging methods, the relevant clinical history and the patient's signs and symptoms.

The goals of the intense and prolonged training and experience for all such imaging experts thus include:

- First, to know what is normal, the spectrum of normal variation and how to distinguish normal from abnormal
- Second, to see and learn a myriad of different appearances of many diseases and to appreciate how they differ from each other.
- Third, to develop a personal internalised image library and knowledge base for each disease entity in the list and its specific features that distinguish it from other similar conditions
- Fourth, to utilise specific imaging techniques that can help to distinguish a one process from another – this is particularly relevant for MRI and nuclear imaging
- Finally, to learn the systematic process of feature analysis and diagnostic convergence that enables the specialist to rapidly discard all diagnoses that do not match key criteria found in that patient, and to narrow in on ideally one or perhaps a very small number of probable diagnoses.

Radiologists are thus operating on the basis of highly empirically derived maxims, strengthened by acquired wisdom and experience that has been codified in a systematic but not intuitive manner. The "truth" in radiology arises from the strength of observation and the use of "gold standards" such as laboratory tests (that may for example confirm an adrenal mass to be a phaechromocytoma that secretes excessive amounts of adrenaline and noradrenaline into the bloodstream), or surgical pathology (where biopsy or excision of a lump may confirm that it does indeed contain cartilage, or infection, or a specific type of cancer). Sometimes it derives from sequential observation in the same patient; a disease that may have been confused with another reveals its true nature with the passage of time – thus a focal haemorrhage in the brain may be seen to involute totally over a few months (which we would expect of a so-called "simple" haemorrhage) or may alternatively develop a focal soft tissue mass, which would declare the underlying cause of the bleed to be due to a brain tumour.

Although radiologists and other imaging practitioners have developed their own systems for epistemological understanding of truth in imaging, they lack any sort of formal grounding in philosophy to truly appreciate the fragility of such truth. The imaging literature is replete with examples of conditions that defy the usual descriptions, or that behave in ways that are not commonly recognised, or that mimic conditions in a manner not previously described. When pressed, most radiologists will admit to these problems and an enlightened few will even go so far as to acknowledge that they are strongly guided by probability in choosing one diagnosis over another. As one imaging adage states, "common things occur commonly", and this proves true, not surprisingly, most of the time. However, exceptions abound, and there are many pitfalls awaiting the unwary diagnostician.

Furthermore, this highly practical and empirical training and experience does little for the radiologist in terms of appreciating clinical ethics and the rights of the patient in day to day practice. In general, radiologists function mostly as the "doctor's doctor", that is they are asked by other doctors to perform a test on a third party, the patient. The patient is generally poorly informed as to the nature, reasons, complexities, pitfalls and risks of the test, and in almost all cases, the radiologist does little to improve the patient's knowledge unless an invasive procedure that carries a significant risk of injury (e. g., angiography), or one that carries great potential medicolegal import (e. g., foetal MRI) is to be performed. Although radiologists have argued for years that they should be treated as consultants, should help guide clinicians in their selection of imaging test and should be the advocates of the patient to decide if an imaging test is likely to be of any value, the reality is that the overwhelming majority of imaging tests requested (or "ordered", as non-radiologists like to say), are performed without any direct questioning or consultation with the radiologists. This is highly pragmatic of course, for the amount of discussion and debate required for each and every imaging test would require hiring additional highly skilled staff to assist in the task (with a very low probability that such tests would be either prevented or altered). Furthermore, for the vast majority of diagnostic tests, the risk to the patient of having the test is extremely low – of the order of 1 in 10,000 to 1 in 200,000 of incurring any sort of significant injury directly as a result of the imaging test. The risks of misinterpretation or miscommunication are many orders of magnitude greater than the test itself. Furthermore, in many societies imaging is dependent for its growth and development on ever-rising workloads and revenues; there are thus many counteracting reasons for imaging specialists to *not* actively pursue the rights of the patient and the appropriateness of the imaging investigation in every case.

It is apparent then that the teaching of philosophy in medical imaging has great potential value – not only for clinical ethics, which is the most obvious application, but also so that radiologists understand the nature, strengths and weaknesses of the system of "truth" that they function under every day. Medical imaging, more than any other discipline of medicine, is highly dependent on the efficiencies of a highly ordered empirical construct of truth in order to function efficiently. But over-reliance on this construct will and does lead to errors in interpretation and diagnosis on a daily basis.

CONCLUSIONS

To conclude then, I hope to have demonstrated that modern medical imaging is complex, rich, multifaceted and advancing at a breathtaking and sometimes overwhelming pace. The collaboration between scientists, imaging experts and other clinical practitioners has driven innovation and development across the entire spectrum of established imaging modalities, with many further developments still to come.

With such rapid advances, it has been difficult for radiologists to adequately contemplate the philosophical underpinnings of their craft. The explosion of new knowledge that accompanies the development of each new imaging method requires integration with the existing knowledge base and a new epistemological understanding based on clinical outcomes, surgical pathology and research. The radiologist by and large still functions at a level of complex pattern recognition intertwined inextricably with a deep knowledge of anatomy, physiology, pathology, clinical medicine and received wisdom in the form of gamuts and differential diagnoses handed down by preceding generations of radiologists.

In this maelstrom of complex and rapid expansion and development of medical imaging, it is clear that the practice paradigm of the past – unquestioned performance of ordered medical imaging tests, with little regard to the patient's needs or rights – needs further enquiry, investigation and change.

It is undeniable that the ever-increasing use of imaging for sometimes smaller and smaller gains, the progressive abstraction of the medical image and its concomitant increasing importance in clinical diagnosis and treatment almost demand that philosophical issues in imaging are studied in much greater detail. I hope that this field will grow and flourish in response to this need.

REFERENCES

Andriole KP, Wolfe JM, Khorasani R, Treves ST, Getty DJ, Jacobson FL, Steigner ML, Pan JJ, Sitek A, Seltzer SE (2011). Optimizing Analysis, Visualization, and Navigation of Large Image Data Sets: One 5000-Section CT Scan Can Ruin Your Whole Day. *Radiology,* 259(2): 346–62.

Anger HO (1953). A multiple scintillation counter *in vivo* scanner. *Am J Roentgenol Radium Ther Nucl Med.* 70: 605–612.

Cho, ZH, Eriksson L, Chan JK (1975). A circular ring transverse axial positron camera in *Reconstruction Tomography in Diagnostic Radiology and Nuclear Medicine*, Ter-Pogossian MM, *Editor.* University Park Press: Baltimore.

Damadian, R. V. (1971). Tumor detection by nuclear magnetic resonance. *Science,* 171: 1151–1153

Damadian, R. V. (1974). Apparatus and method for detecting cancer in tissue. *US Patent 3,789,832*

Do T, Wan C-N, Casella V, Fowler JS, Wolf AP, Reivich M, Kuhl DE (1978). Labeled 2-deoxy-D-glucose analogs. -labeled 2-deoxy-2-fluoro-D-glucose, 2-deoxy-2-fluoro-D-mannose and C-14-2-deoxy-2-fluoro-D-glucose, *The Journal of Labelled Compounds and Radiopharmaceuticals.* 14: 175–182.

Donald I, Macvicar J, Brown TG (1958). Investigation of Abdominal Masses by Pulsed Ultrasound. *The Lancet,* 271: 1188–1195.

Filler, A. G. (2009). The History, Development and Impact of Computed Imaging in Neurological Diagnosis and Neurosurgery: CT, MRI, and DTI. *Nature Precedings.* URL: http://precedings. nature.com/documents/3267/version/4/html. Accessed 2 June 2011.

Hounsfield, G. N. (1973). Computerized transverse axial scanning (tomography). 1. Description of system. *The British Journal of Radiology.* 46(552): 1016–22.

Kossoff, G., Garrett, W. J., and Radovanovich, G. (1973) Gray scale echography in obstetrics and gynaecology. *Commonwealth Acoustic Laboratories, Report No. 59, Sydney, Australia.*

Johnson KM, Dennis JM, Dowe DA (2010). Extracardiac findings on coronary CT angiograms: Limited versus complete image review. *AJR Am J Roentgenol.* 195(1): 143–8.

Kelly WM, Kucharczyk W, Kucharczyk J, Kjos B, Peck WW, Norman D, Newton TH (1988). Posterior pituitary ectopia: an MR feature of pituitary dwarfism. *AJNR Am J Neuroradiol.* 9(3): 453–60.

Kemerink M, Dierichs TJ, Dierichs J, Huynen HJ, Wildberger JE, van Engelshoven JM, Kemerink GJ (2011). Characteristics of a first-generation x-ray system. *Radiology,* 259(2): 534–9.

Lauterbur, P. C. (1973). Image formation by induced local interactions: examples employing nuclear magnetic resonance. *Nature,* 242: 190.

Mancini DM, Bolinger L, Li H, Kendrick K, Chance B, Wilson JR (1994). Validation of near-infrared spectroscopy in humans. *Journal of Applied Physiology* 77(6): 2740–2747.

Mercuri E, Bushby K, Ricci E, Birchall D, Pane M, Kinali M, Allsop J, Nigro V, Sáenz A, Nascimbeni A, Fulizio L, Angelini C, Muntoni F (2005). Muscle MRI findings in patients with limb girdle muscular dystrophy with calpain 3 deficiency (LGMD2A) and early contractures. *Neuromuscular Disorders.* 15(2): 164–71.

Newman PG & Rozycki GS (1998). The history of ultrasound. *Surgical Clinics of North America,* 78(2): 178–195.

"The Nobel Prize in Physics 1904". Nobelprize.org. 3 Jun 2011. URL: http://nobelprize.org/nobel_prizes/physics/laureates/1904/. Accessed 2 June 2011.

Ogawa, S., Lee, T. M., Kay, A. R., & Tank, D. W. (1990). Brain magnetic resonance imaging with contrast dependent on blood oxygenation. *Proceedings of the National Academy of Sciences of the United States of America,* 87(24): 9868–72.

Robertson JS, Marr RB, Rosenblum M, Radeka V, Yamamoto YL (1973). 32-Crystal positron transverse section detector, in *Tomographic Imaging in Nuclear Medicine*, Freedman GS, *Editor.* The Society of Nuclear Medicine: New York. pp. 142–153.

Röntgen, W. K. (1895). Über eine neue Art von Strahlen ("On A New Kind Of Rays"). *Sitzungsberichte der Physikalisch-Medizinischen Gesellschaft in Würzburg*, 1895, Band 137, S. 132–141.

Rossoff M (2008). How the Beatles funded the CT scan. *CNET*, July 21, 2008 11:07 AM PDT. URL: http://news.cnet.com/8301-13526_3-9995690-27.html. Accessed April 10, 2011.

Slowiczek F and Peters PM. The Discovery Of Radioactivity: The Dawn of the Nuclear Age. *Access Excellence Classic Collection, Physics.org*. URL: http://www.physics.org/explorelink.asp?id= 568&q=path&currentpage=1&age=0&knowledge=0&item=9. Accessed April 2, 2011.

The History of Ultrasound: A collection of recollections, articles, interviews and images. *www.ob-gyn.net*, URL: http://www.obgyn.net/ultrasound/ultrasound.asp?page=/us/news_articles/ultra-sound_history/asp-history-toc. Retrieved December 1, 2010.

Woo, J. (2002) A short history of the development of ultrasound in obstetrics and gynecology, part 2. *www.obgyn.net*, URL: http://www.ob-ultrasound.net/history2.html. Retrieved December 1, 2010.

Yodh A, Chance B (1995). Spectroscopy and imaging with diffusing light. *Physics Today*, March issue, pp 34–40.

II. IMAGING:
ONTOLOGY AND TRUTH IN REPRESENTATION

MEDICAL IMAGING:
PICTURES, "AS IF" AND THE POWER OF EVIDENCE[1]

Irmgard Müller, Heiner Fangerau

ABSTRACT

Contemporary medical practices are impossible without imaging techniques. One example is the practice of neuroimaging. Current literature in the scope of "Medicine Studies" has highlighted the "Gestaltsehen" perspective and has discussed the process of creating visual evidence using complex combinations of numerical methods, statistical procedures and visualization-algorithms. In line with this research, this special issue of Medicine Studies focuses – using different examples – on the specific use of visualizations, the transformation of observations and data into images, the shift in medical viewing patterns caused by new visualization techniques and the nomothetic function of visual discourse networks for distinguishing the normal and the pathological.

In the history of medicine, analyses focusing on the epistemic status of a "reality" or "visibility" produced by measurement and evaluation are a desideratum along with studies on the evidentiary value of technically evoked images. Consequently, the topic of this editorial is the epistemological potential of images and artifacts in medicine. By providing two examples from the history of medicine (Paul Ehrlich's images of the side chain theory and images from sperms), we will examine the claim of evidence put forward by scientists with the help of visualizations. The "as if"-status (following the philosopher Hans Vaihinger) of images in Medicine is discussed.

A TIME OF ICONOGRAPHY

There is no doubt that we are living in a time of iconography. Pictures and images surround us from birth until death. Throughout our whole lives (and even before birth and after death) we are the product and the producer of a pure flood of images, which determine our thinking, wishes and imagination. The omnipresence of images is the result of a fundamental shift during modernity in both the status and modalities of presentation procedures. The concomitant increase in technical methods for image production resulted in a new kind of knowledge formation compared

---

1   This is a revised version of an article which appeared under the same title as the editorial for a special issue of the journal "Medicine Studies" published by Springer.

to premodern times. It is a specific element of these modern and postmodern processes of knowledge formation and dissemination that knowledge itself seems to be more dependent on the possibilities of its illustration, demonstration, and presentation than on the matter or cause itself. Nevertheless, regarding the "claim for truth," this practice is not less unproblematic than knowledge that comes along without any form of representation.[2]

Contemporary medical practices are impossible without imaging techniques. Whereas in many disciplines the history and philosophy of visual culture plays an important role (Lynch 2006), in medicine only single aspects have been highlighted so far. One example is the practice of neuroimaging (cf. (Dijck 2005)). The "Gestaltsehen" perspective has been highlighted (Burri 2008, 214) and the process of creating visual evidence using complex combinations of numerical methods, statistical procedures and visualization-algorithms has been discussed previously (Schinzel 2006; Huber 2009). In line with this research, this conference volume of the 1st conference on Medical Imaging held in Ulm in 2010 focuses on the specific use of visualizations, the transformation of observations and data into images, the shift in medical viewing patterns caused by new visualization techniques and the nomothetic function of visual discourse networks for distinguishing the normal and the pathological.

The conference proceedings intend to stimulate further debates and research. For example, we lack systematic studies regarding the transformation and modeling of medical data by evaluation, selection and statistical processing, which are not only phenomena of the computer age but have existed long before. From the existing literature and papers in this issue, it is clear that questions regarding the validity of medical images are of special interest: Many modern visualization techniques do not refer to observable correlates but to complex mathematical processing procedures, which have caused a paradoxical phenomenon, since they produce virtual images that do not exist as visible entities (Adelmann, Frercks et al. 2009). In the history of medicine, analyses focusing on the epistemic status of a "reality" or "visibility" produced by measurement and evaluation are a desideratum along with studies on the evidentiary value of technically evoked images. Consequently, the topic of this editorial is the epistemological potential of images and artifacts in medicine. By providing two examples from the history of medicine, we will examine the claim of evidence put forward by scientists with the help of visualizations. These visualizations are scientific pictures, which are the result of the interaction of processing measured data, picture creation, amplification and reduction, and human interpretation.

---

2   The body of literature regarding the practice of visualization is steadily increasing. An instructive bibliographic essay review is offered by Monika Dommann (Dommann 2004).

PAUL EHRLICH'S IMAGES

The first example involves Paul Ehrlich's central contribution to immunology – the side-chain theory. Cambrosio, Jacobi and Keating have shown that the development, reception and acceptance of Ehrlich's side-chain theory, which explained the immune response as an antibody- receptor reaction, offers an illuminating example of the role and function of graphical images during the implementation of a medical theory (Cambrosio, Jacobi et al. 1993). Ehrlich based his side-chain theory on his earlier systematic studies on the relationship between the chemical structures of pharmaceuticals and their distribution in different organs (Ehrlich 1901) and the research for his habilitation, in which he had examined the organism's need for oxygen (Ehrlich 1885).[3] The underlying idea of his working hypothesis can be summarized as follows: living cells have side chains on their surfaces similar to those of the benzene ring, which can link with toxins (e. g., from bacteria) and make these toxins innoxious. Since the receptiveness of an organism for toxins depended on these "protoplasm groups", he named them receptors. Ehrlich imagined the process of "detoxification" as a chemical reaction similar to the neutralization of an acid by a base.

According to Ehrlich's experimentally supported view, each receptor could only react with specific agents depending on its chemical structure. The toxins had to fit in the receptor like a key in a lock, an analogy which was coined by the chemist Emil Fischer in 1894 to describe the stereochemical anchoring of enzyme-substrate-binding (Fischer 1894). Ehrlich used this stereochemical conception as an explanation for the antitoxin doctrine he developed while studying diphtheria toxin and diphtheria antitoxin. He attributed specific groups of atoms to both reacting agents (toxin and antitoxin) in the process of detoxification. He assumed that the toxin consisted of two chemically different parts. One part of the toxin, which linked to the side-chain of the cell's protoplasm,[4] was called the haptophore group, and the second part carrying the poison was called the toxophore group (Ehrlich 1904). If the haptophore group bound to the cell's receptor, then the receptor switched off. Ehrlich theorized that the cell tried to repair this defect by regenerating and releasing the same specific group of molecules in excess to replenish their circulation in the blood. Now the receptors as antibodies could intercept and render the intruding toxins harmless.

Ehrlich formulated this audacious and complex explanation of the mysterious processes of immunity in 1897 after performing experiments in animals with ricin and antiricin (Ehrlich 1897; Ehrlich 1897). At first, his theory was disputed. Ehrlich himself encountered repeated difficulties because the results of his animal experiments were instable. In a letter to his cousin Karl Weigert, a professor of pathology

3   On the history of the side chain theory see (Silverstein 1989; Silverstein 2002).
4   Ehrlich at first followed the terminology of benzole chemistry and called the binding groups of the cell protoplasmatic "side chains". Later he used the term "receptor", because the term "side chain" insinuated far too simple concepts regarding their structure (Ehrlich and Morgenroth 1904).

in Frankfurt, Ehrlich lamented at the end of December 1896: "Here everything is fluctuating and it is, as if one tried to build a palace in the swamps. After all it eventually works, but it costs a dreadful lot of animals, anger and boredom" (Heymann 1928).[5] In their correspondence, Ehrlich expressed admiration for Weigert for his mastery of staining techniques, and Weigert critically commented on Ehrlich's experiments. This correspondence also reveals the first graphical representation of the events Ehrlich assumed were taking place on the cellular level. In 1898, Ehrlich cursorily sketched the processes to foster understanding of his theory, and he commented on his picture not without self-mockery with the concomitant question "beautiful representations?" ("Schöne Figuren?").

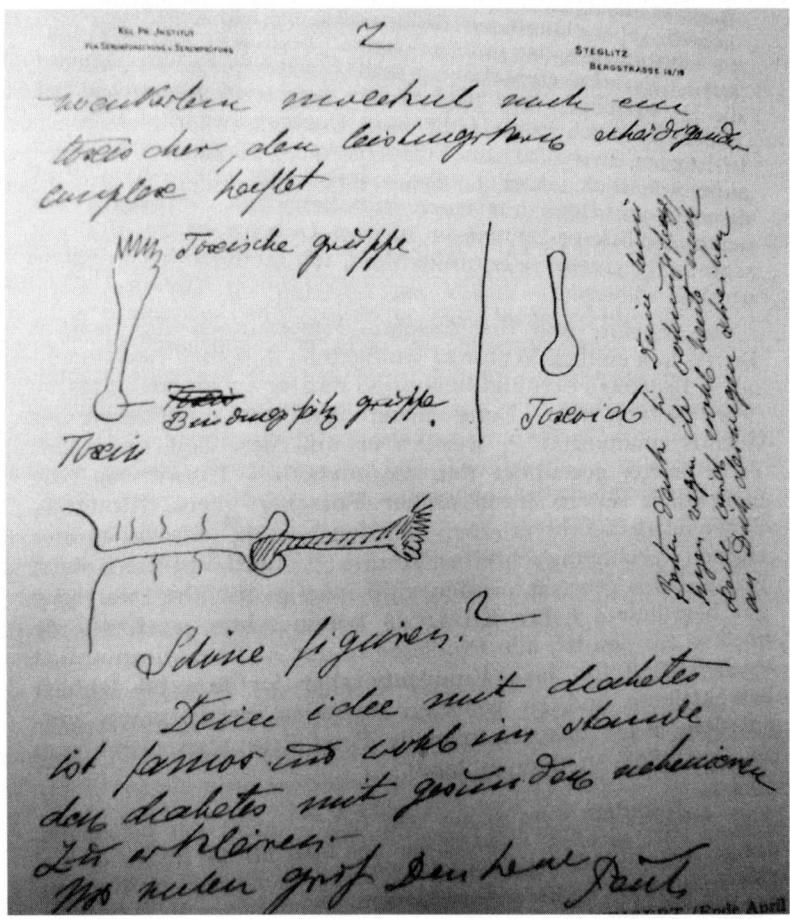

Fig. 1: Letter of Paul Ehrlich mit "Schönen Figuren" First sketch of the side chain theory in a letter from Paul Ehrlichs to Carl Weigert. In: Paul Heymann, Zur Geschichte der Seitenkettentheorie Paul Ehrlichs. Klinische Wochenschrift, Bd. 7 (1928) S. 1307

5   This and all of the following translations from German by HF.

Ehrlich's sketch shows that he considered the binding of toxins by the cell's protoplasm as analogous to the physiological nutrition of the cell. Soon after, Ehrlich explicitly stated that there was a similarity between toxins and food molecules when he declared: "The toxins, as highly complicated products of herbal and animal cells, share certain haptophore groups with food molecules and are consequently anchored by appropriate receptors of the protoplasm as well" (Ehrlich and Morgenroth 1904).

Ehrlich's ambiguous signature "beautiful representations" was chosen by Cambrosio, Jacobi and Keating in a similar translation as the title for their "beautiful pictures" essay mentioned above (Cambrosio, Jacobi et al. 1993). In this essay, they examined how Ehrlich developed diagrams from his first sketch to implement his hypothesis. Our following remarks are based on their findings.

Two years after his sketch of the "beautiful representations" in his letter to Weigert, Ehrlich published the first diagrams to depict his theory of immunity. These images were added to the printed version of an invited lecture Ehrlich gave in London for the Royal Society (Ehrlich 1900). In this paper two images appeared for the first time, which in the following years were modified, refined and combined to larger complexes. As the levels of the single components' abstraction increased, the specificity of the functions they represented grew. When the side chain theory was applied to explain haematolysis, both the receptor apparatuses and the number of assumed immune bodies were duplicated. Ehrlich conceptualized that an amboceptor circulated in the blood with two different haptophoric groups, which acted as an intermediate between the erythrocytes and complement (Ehrlich and Morgenroth 1900). Soon Ehrlich's scheme did not only operate with receptors of a first, second or third order, but it also included manifold complements, toxoids, toxonoids, toxons, complementoids, epitoxoids, and nutriceptors.[6]

At first, Ehrlich abstained from giving chemical definitions or clear statements regarding the chemical existence or non-existence of these agents. In his London lecture, he emphasized that his figures were hypothetical in character. He explicitly declared that his diagrams should be looked at without any morphological considerations. Ehrlich emphasized that they were only a pictorial method of displaying and explaining his views about the metabolism of the cell and the way that toxins and antitoxins acted during immunization.

Despite of Ehrlich's introductory remarks concerning the visualization of his theory of immunization in which he saw nothing more than "the clearly arranged abstraction of an experience gained from an extraordinary large number of exact experiments" (Ehrlich 1904, V), his diagrams did not fail to have an impact. They suggested and provoked the impression of a real fact. In particular, the ostensive visualization of the single components, which resembled living organisms, seemed to confirm the belief that he had been able to unravel the mystery of life. Ehrlich presented structures with tentacles stemming from the protoplasm to represent the associations of polyps. His images resembled for example those of polyps and medusa published by Gegenbaur (Gegenbaur 1854).

---

6   See the compilation by Schatiloff (Schatiloff 1908, 9 ff.).

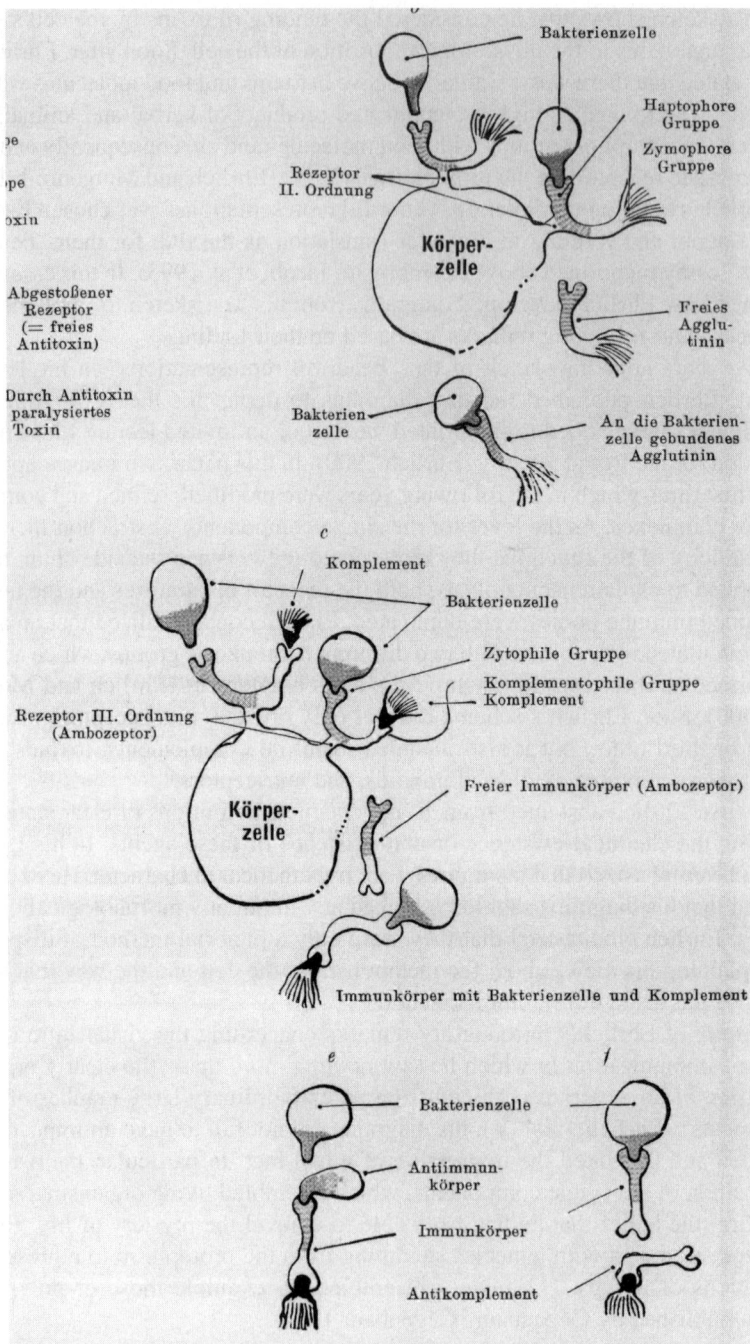

Fig. 2: Receptors of the 2nd and 3rd order after drawings by Paul Ehrlich. From: Handbuch der pathogenen Mikroorganismen, 1904

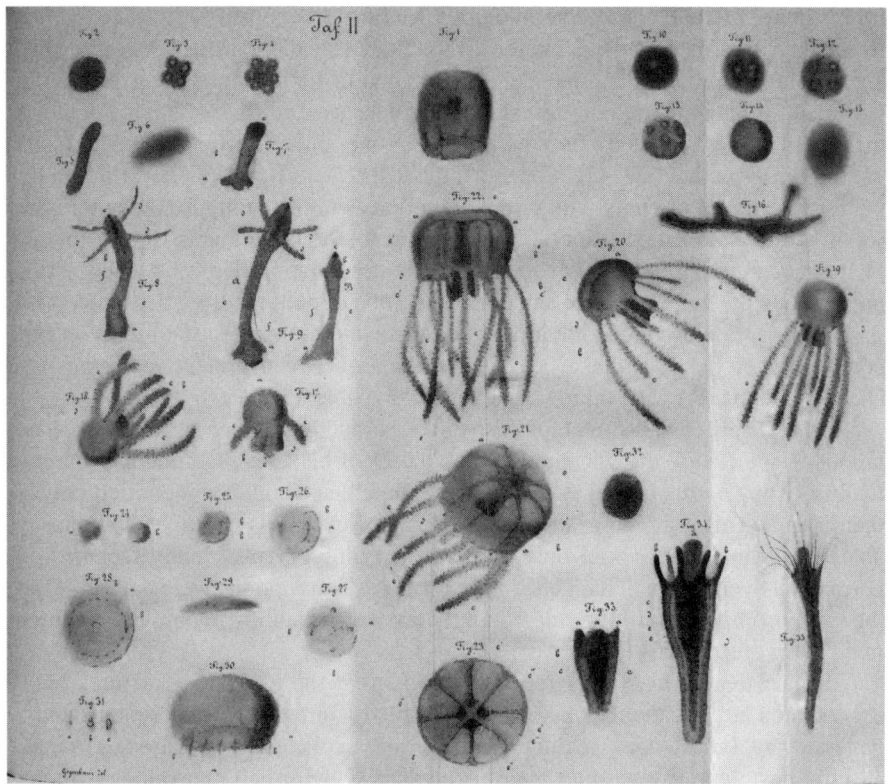

Figure 3: Developmental stages of Polyps.
From: Gegenbaur, Zur Lehre von Generationswechsel und Fortpflanzung
von Medusen und Polypen. Wiesbaden 1854

Later Ehrlich also used analogies from botany. The visitors to his institute, who had wished to see cell receptors through his microscope, were deeply disappointed when they were only shown these symbols instead of reality (Cambrosio, Jacobi et al. 1993).

Ehrlich's theory was rapidly disseminated not only because of the analogies in his graphical representations, but also due to his illustrative textual presentation. By extensively using metaphors and analogies, Ehrlich intensified the impression that he was describing reactions of real, existing chemical bodies, which anchored and captured toxins like fishing rods and snapped poisonous elements up with the help of their tentacles.[7] Ehrlich received admiration, but also faced some severe criticisms

---

7   As an example may serve Ehrlich's essay on the theory of lysin's actions, in which he described the assimilation of giant molecules in the cell (Ehrlich 1899): "In sehr zweckmäßiger Weise wird solches erreicht werden können, wenn der Fangarm des Protoplasmas zu gleicher Zeit als Träger einer fermentativen Gruppe diese sofort in nahe räumliche Beziehung zu der zu verdau-

for his images. The French bacteriologist Jules Bordet vehemently attacked Ehrlich. Bordet had described non-specific serum components – the so called alexines, which correspond with today's complement system, and in 1919, Bordet received the Nobel Prize for his immunologic research. Bordet accused Ehrlich of having achieved the acceptance of his theory only with the help of popular illustrations in the mould of children's' picture books (Christ and Tauber 1997). In Bordet's view, Ehrlich had put forward his theory only with visual definitions without caring for the ontological status of the assumed substances. Bordet himself strictly abstained from using any pictorial representation and advocated textual presentation. He considered textual presentation the more adequate and precise method of putting forward a theory. Similarly, other scientists argued that the diagrams were too imprecise to represent the complexity of the protoplasm and the reactions between protein molecules and chemical atoms that were taking place on the invisible level.

Indeed, Ehrlich had aimed for this vagueness and indefiniteness in his representations. He was sure that the single components of his side-chain theory were not really existing entities. They were obviously unreal and could be identified only by their assumed effects. Their factual existence, however, was unproven and unprovable. The components could only be discerned through consistently repeated experimental events, which happened as if Ehrlich's assumptions were correct. Thus, the single components of the side-chain theory were scientific fiction, not a copy of reality (Dworetzky 1914).

Ehrlich treated his visual representations as if the assumed structures really existed, and he used them as heuristic tools to structure further experiments and to generate new knowledge. He did not use them as explications of causes or to make specific postulations regarding their appearance. For Ehrlich, the value of his images materialized in a constructive alternativism, in their status of images that represented his side-chain theory "as if" its postulated elements existed in real. Their power as a model was achieved through their plausibility and the sensation of evidence they emanated at first sight. However, the "epistemic power of representativeness", using Sybille Kraemer's (Krämer 2009, 12) terminology, turned out to be fallacious, since it did not lead to the actual chemical reality.[8] Ehrlich's visualiza-

---

enden und zu assimilierenden Beute bringt. Derartige zweckmäßige Einrichtungen, dass der Fangapparat zugleich verdauende Wirkung ausübt, finden wir ja in der ganzen Reihe der verdauenden höheren Pflanzen in der verschiedensten Art und Form. So sezernieren die Tentakeln der Drosera, also Fangarme im allergröbsten Sinne, die das gefangene Object umgeben, eine Flüssigkeit, die stark verdauende Wirkung ausübt. [...] Wir nehmen also an, dass bei der Ergreifung dieser [Toxine] und anderer hochcomplicirter Körper Seitenketten besonderer Art vorhanden sind, die ausser dem fangenden Complex noch einen anderen Complex enthalten, der durch Fixation geeigneter Fermente Verdauungswirkung auslösen kann. [...]".

8   Ehrlich himself closed his introduction into the side chain theory stressing the heuristic power of the combination of single research results and the principles of his theory: "Die unübersehbare Fülle der Einzelthatsachen läßt sich ohne Zwang in die hier kurz dargestellten Prinzipien [der Seitenkettentheorie] einordnen, die zugleich heuristische Kraft genug bewähren, um ihrerseits wieder zur Auffindung zahlreicher neuer experimenteller Thatsachen zu führen" (Ehrlich and Morgenroth 1904).

tions reminded his viewers of living organisms and could be related to well-known examples, such as the old conception of the body as an organism that is ready to battle hostile agents. This immediacy secured his pictures and the theory they represented a lasting impact, which was independent of their real ontological status. Ludwik Fleck coined the terms "collective thought style" and "thought coercion" to describe this type of directed perception, which goes hand in hand with an according theoretical and factual processing of what is perceived (Fleck 1980). With regard to Ehrlich, one might postulate that "vision coercion" and diagrammatic coercion could explain the evidentiary power of his images.

A glance into a modern immunology textbook reveals that the immunologic diagrams put forward by Ehrlich to visualize unknown immune system events still claim validity. Furthermore, they still appear to encapsulate and reproduce real structures (e. g. Murphy, Travers et al. 2009).

IMAGING SPERMS AND CONCEPTS
OF EMBRYOLOGICAL DEVELOPMENT

A second illustrative example of this general principle of filtering an observer's perception is the debate that occurred during the 17th and 18th centuries among reproductive biologists. Here again, theoretical conceptions evoked observations and illustrations, which retroacted with the underlying idea. At the time, few questions preoccupied scientists as much as those involving human development, and few debates challenged the existing metaphysical world order to such an extent as these questions.

In 1651, William Harvey published his observation that embryonic development originated from the egg, which led to a scientific dispute (Harvey 1651). His dictum "omne vivum ex ovo" challenged the classic doctrine of spontaneous generation of living beings from inorganic material. Since Harvey was unable to describe the role of sperm in generation, his dictum also challenged the validity of the theory that female and male sperm contributed equally to human development. No matter how hard Harvey tried, he could not detect any sperm in the uteri of his dissected research animals (Goltz 1986). He concluded that male sperm stimulated the egg through an immaterial "aura seminalis" (cf. Schurig 1720), a theory, which did not convince his contemporaries. Although Harvey was highly regarded as a scientific authority, since he had described the circulation of blood, his tenets on human development were severely criticized.

Scientists began intensive investigations into the field of human development. After 20 years of thorough research, it caused a sensation when the first spermatozoa were sighted under the microscope. The spermatozoa were pictured as small animalcula – real creatures with heads and tails. The paradox powers postulated by Harvey seemed to have materialized. The first image of this mysterious animal appeared on the margins of a writing of the Dutch physicist Nicolas Hartsoeker (1656–1725) to Christian Huyghens (Huyghens 1899, 58–61). Hartsoeker reported in his letter and in print (Hartsoeker 1678, 355–366) that he had observed uncountable small creatures, which resembled small eels or tadpoles in a cockerel's sperm under the microscope. Sixteen years later he reprinted his spermatic animals in a book on optics with the remark that human sperm looked the same (Hartsoeker 1694, 227). He added that each sperm included a female and a male exemplar, which was inserted into the egg in order to grow and to be nurtured here. To emphasize this textually presented idea, he added a microscopic view showing a spermatic animal that appeared as a cowering homunculus. The long tail housed the allantoic vein to allow for placental nidation. However, Hartsoeker was very careful regarding the real existence of these embryological beings. When he later copied this picture in other works, the original explanatory function of the image was blended with empirical observations. It became "real".

Even more spectacular was the image of a spermatic animal published by the secretary of the Academy of Montpellier Francois Plantade under the anagram Dalenpatius. Dalenpatius claimed to have observed the moult of a spermatozoon under the microscope (Dalenpatius [= Francois Plantade] 1699–1700). As proof, he added an image of a moulting homunculus whose head, breast, arms and legs were still mantled with an outer skin. The credibility of this report was highly questioned. The French physician Jean Astruc could only interpret the image as a satire put forward by Dalenpatius to ridicule preformationists who believed that the forms of living beings preexisted in miniature versions (Astruc 1740, 1002 f.). Nevertheless, the image had a lasting effect. It suited preformationism so perfectly that in 1721 the Italian biologist Antonio Vallisneri did not hesitate to include a reproduction of these animalcules in a table of known spermatozoons (Vallisneri 1721, Table I, Figure 7–9 and p. 6–7).

No matter how unusual these fantastic images might appear to us today, when they were published in the 17th century they seemed to fit the expectations of biologists who were using microscopes to visualize the invisible. For instance, in Francesco Redi's representations of fishworms, he attributed them with a human shape (Redi 1684, Table 23). Another example is Joblot's descriptions of the organisms he observed in an extraction of anemones (Joblot 1718, p. 58, Table 56, Figure 12). He described that the back of one six-legged animal was covered with a mask resembling a human face. Perhaps Joblot was ridiculing microscopic representation practices, but the basis of this image may have been more credible. Modern representations of hydrachnidia still have some similarities to Jablot's image (Kaestner 1969, 777 f.).

Although the pioneer of microscopic research and sperm visualization Antonj van Leeuwenhoek rejected and criticized these exaggerated visual interpretations (Leeuwenhoek 1719, 82–94), he contributed his own interpretations of microscopic images. In many works Leeuwenhoek described vivid, visible structures and vessels inside the animalcula (Leeuwenhoek 1678, Table 13). He also promoted the idea that organisms and their body parts were preformed in the spermatic animals. His visualizations helped to fix and implement the preformistic ideas (Vallisneri 1721, Table I).[9]

---

9   Vallisneri combines images of spermatic animals following the descriptions of Leeuwenhoek, Nicolas Andry and Dalenpatius. He adds the comment that it is impossible to neglect the factual existence of the imaged animals (una cosa di fatto) facing so many prominent witnesses.

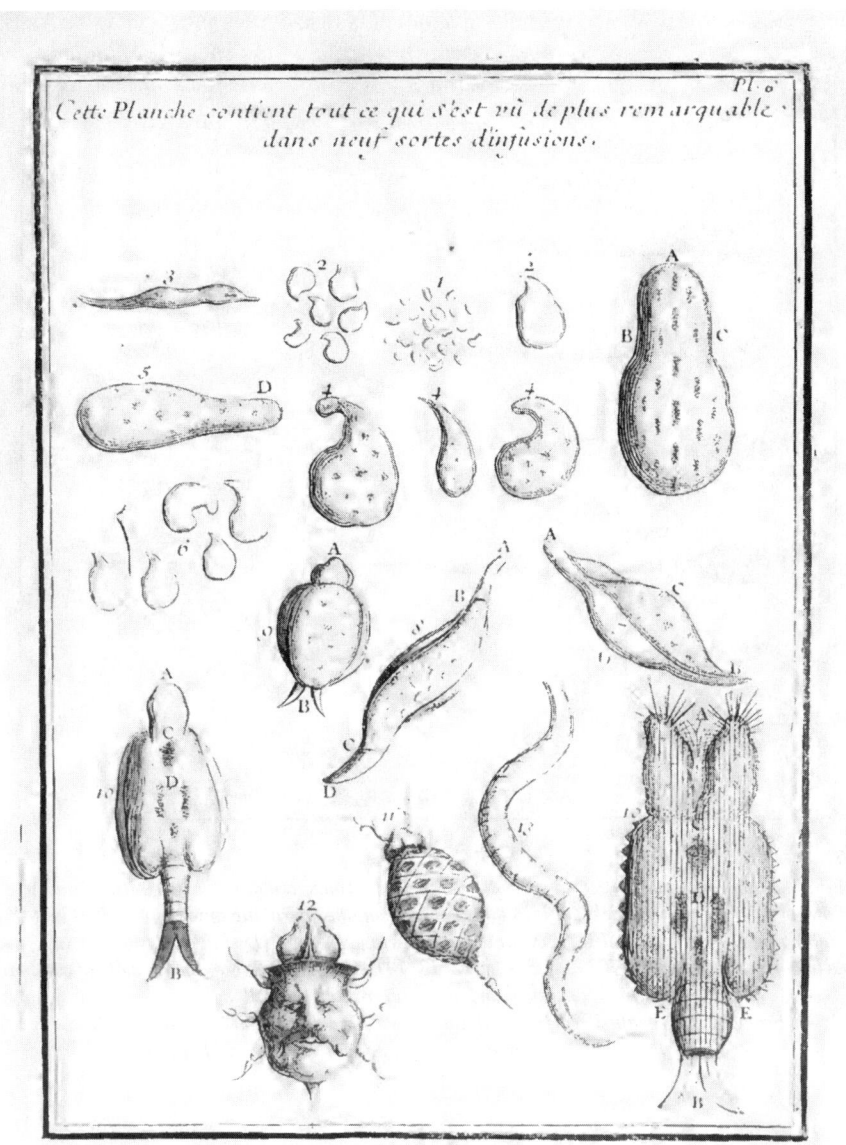

Fig. 4: Organisms found in an infusion of anemones described by Joblot.
"Tout le dessus de son corps est couvert d'un beau masque bien formé, de figure humaine,
parfaitement bien fait; comme on en peut juger par ce dessein, où l'on voit six pattes et une queuë,
sortant de dessous ce masque, qui est couronne d'une coëffure singuliere" (S. 57f.)
From Joblot, J.: Descriptions et usages de plusieurs nouveaux microscopes,
tant simples que composez. Paris 1718, Taf. 6, Fig. 12

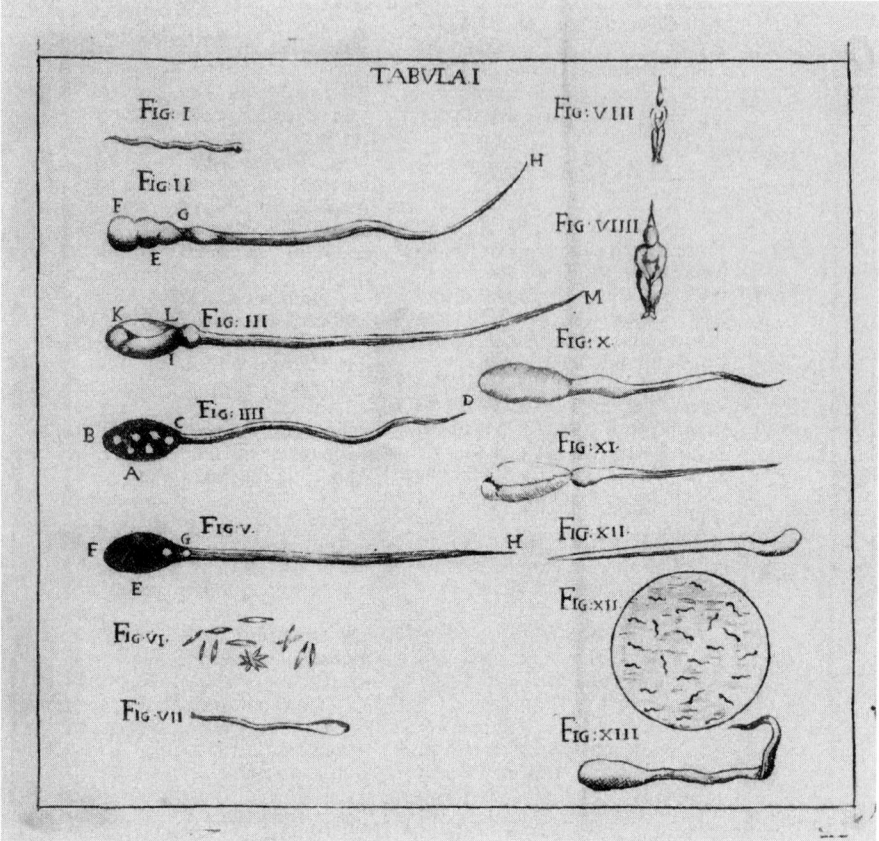

Fig. 5: Plate displaying different spermatic animals (vermi spermatici): Fig. II, III, IV and V following A. van Leeuwenhoek; – Fig. VI (salt crystals in the spermatic animal), VII, VIII und IX following Dalenpatius; – Fig. X, XI and XII following N. Andry (De la génération des vers dans le corps de l'homme, 1701, Taf. 3, Fig. 12, 13, 14); – Fig. XIII Spermatic animals of a rabbit in motion, observed under the microscope by Vallisneri.
From: Antonio Vallisneri: Istoria della generazione dell'uomo, e degli animali, se sia d'vermicelli spermatici, o dalle uoava. Venedig 1721, Taf. I

Leeuwenhoek's authority as the inventor of the microscope strengthened the validity of his exposures, and his less dramatic visualizations convinced with ostensive precision. These images were carried from handbook to handbook: Even 150 years later, the impact of Leeuwenhoek's images lasted on. In 1821, Prevost and Dumas described the origin of sperm in the testicles, which contradicted the prevailing idea that spermatozoa could be classified as independent organisms (Prévost and Dumas 1821–1822, Table 1–2). Nevertheless, their illustrations referred to Leuwenhoek. The idea that spermatozoa were organisms was bound to contemporary thinking to such an extent that in 1837 the physiologist Gustav Valentin described the mouth, anus, stomach and early stages of evolutionary development in bear sperm (Valentin 1837, Table 24).

After Leeuwenhoek's first description of sperm, spermatogenesis became an important field of research, and Harvey's observation that the egg was the starting point of reproduction was more or less neglected. Only a few ovulists challenged the tenets of the animalculists. It might be argued that Harvey's abandonment of images hindered the reception of his findings. Except for its allegoric frontispiece, Harvey's work did not contain any figures. Harvey intentionally had abstained from using visualizations as stated in his foreword (Harvey 1651, 10). He distrusted images of any kind because he believed they abstracted, generalized and distorted in contrast to precise observations. Any image could only be a false representation of its object. Harvey believed that only own immediate observations were credible and reliable.

Nevertheless, even if scientists of the 17th and 18th century agreed with Harvey's statement regarding images, they still used visual representations. Their critical use constituted a theory that was then again backed by images. Last but not least, the ovulists and animalculists agreed on one point. Both followed the preformist tradition. Therefore, they both tended to display homunculi in their respective microscopic images, as can be viewed in a 1729 figure by the Dutch scientists Thomas Kerckring (Kerckring 1729).

CONCLUSION

What can be concluded from these examples about the practice of medical imaging and the evidentiary power of pictures? Both examples show that scientific images cannot only be seen as illustrations of experimentally induced or morphological facts. They are bound to scientific practice, the thought styles of a thought collective, the cultures of popularizing knowledge and the cultures of the public understanding of science. Additionally, they are of course constituted by preexisting concepts. They represent the observed objects as if they existed in reality – a practice Immanuel Kant had considered to be not only possible but theoretically and practically necessary when the existing concepts do not suffice to provide explanation and understanding of the unknown (Vaihinger 1911).[10] On this basis, the philosopher Hans Vaihinger established his philosophy of "as if", a fictionalism, which would see the aspect of "as if" in the two examples above instead of empty fiction. As our examples reveal, the "as if" in these cases has its own theoretical and practical value, which leads to theoretical and practical consequences. Thus, the evidence of "as if" images also lies in their power to produce plausible consequences. In a Festschrift for Vaihinger, the system biologist Ludwig von Bertalanffy commented on the meaning of Vaihinger's analogical factionalism stating that every interpreta-

---

10   Prolegomena to Any Future Metaphysics That Will Be Able to Present Itself as a Science
     § 57/58

tion of reality remains a "risky adventure of reason". Either one should generally abstain from interpreting the entity of any object or one should be aware of the fact that these interpretations have the characteristics of an analogy. There is no proof that the "real" world has the same structure as it is attributed by our own experience, analogies and metaphors (Bertalanffy 1986, 86–87).

Established patterns and conventions of perception shape the representation of these analogies in images. They constitute on the one hand how knowledge is displayed and on the other hand direct the formulation and presentation of new knowledge. Only images fitting these traditions can be trusted, and only these images are attributed with some evidentiary power. They are consciously false assumptions put forward for the sake of their functional results. Whoever accepts this character would agree with revisions. As the philosopher Arnold Kowalewski argued, none of these fictions would be privileged, and these (scientific) assumptions – and thus their visual representations – followed the "law of shifting ideas". Whenever the philosophy of "as if" fictionalized certain ideas after critical inquiry, it weakened its impact, but attracted new followers. Consequently, it founded an "image collective" ("Ideengemeinschaft"), a concept later taken up by Ludwik Fleck as the "thought collective" (Kowalewski 1986, 230).

For the history of medical imaging, this theory means that any illustrator has to adapt his visualizations to the vision coercions of the respective thought collective. When illustrations are produced or signed by authorities, this increases their evidentiary power. Citations of these illustrations and re-citations of patterns introduced by these authorities increase the credibility of the respective images. Finally, by reiteration and the solidification of a theory, the original explanatory function of an image can be transformed into an empirical observation. As a consequence the former "as if" status transcends into an "it is" status, which might be deceptive but is taken for reality. The image itself has become the proof. There is no evidentiary power *per se*; there is only a power of evidence, which is constituted by those who produce medical images and negotiate them with their recipients. Thus, the evidentiary power of medical imaging depends on how convincingly the borderline between "as if" and "it is" is transcended. The transition of this borderline is the underlying story of the following papers, which hopefully leads to fruitful further discussions in this journal and beyond.

REFERENCES

Adelmann, R., J. Frercks, et al. (2009). Datenbilder. Zur digitalen Bildpraxis in den Naturwissenschaften. Bielefeld, transcript Verlag.

Astruc, J. (1740). De Morbis Venereis Libri novem. *Editio altera, Tomus II*. Paris.

Bertalanffy, L. v. (1986). Vaihingers Lehre von der analogischen Fiktion in ihrer Bedeutung für die Naturphilosophie. Die Philosophie des Als Ob und das Leben. *Festschrift zu Hans Vaihingers 80. Geburtstag. A. Seidel. Aalen*, Scientia: 82–91.

Burri, R. (2008). Doing Images. *Zur Praxis medizinischer Bilder*. Bielefeld.

Cambrosio, A., D. Jacobi, et al. (1993). *"Ehrlich's "Beautiful Pictures" and the Controversial Beginnings of Immunological Imagery."* Isis 84: 662–699.

Christ, E. and A. Tauber (1997). "Debating Humoral Immunity and Epistemology: The Rivalry of the Immunochemists Jules Bordet and Paul Ehrlich." *Journal of the History of Biology* 30: 321–356.

Dalenpatius [= Francois Plantade] (1699–1700). Extrait d'une Lettre de M. DALENPATIUS à l'Auteur de ces Nouvelles, contenant une découverte curiseuse, faite par le moyen du Microscope. In: *Nouvelles de la République des Lettres*, t. IV: 552–554.

Dijck, J. v. (2005). The transparent body: A cultural analysis of medical imaging. Seattle, *University of Washington Press*.

Dommann, M. (2004). "Vom Bild zum Wissen: eine Bestandsaufnahme wissenschaftshistorischer Bildforschung." *Gesnerus* 61: 77–89.

Dworetzky, A. (1914). "Zur erkenntnistheoretischen Würdigung der Ehrlichschen Seitenkettentheorie." *Deutsche medizinische Wochenschrift* 40: 1324–1326.

Ehrlich, P. (1885). *Das Sauerstoff-Bedürfniss des Organismus. Eine farbenanalytische Studie*. Berlin, Hirschwald.

Ehrlich, P. (1897). "Die Wertbemessung des Diphtherieheilserums und deren theoretische Grundlagen." *Klinisches Jahrbuch* 6: 299–326.

Ehrlich, P. (1897). "Zur Kenntnis der Antitoxinwirkung." *Fortschritte der Medicin* 15/2: 41–43.

Ehrlich, P. (1899). "Zur Theorie der Lysinwirkung." *Berliner Klinische Wochenschrift*: 6–9.

Ehrlich, P. (1900). "Croonian lecture: On Immunity with special Reference to Cell Life." *Proceedings of the Royal Society of London* 66: 424–448.

Ehrlich, P. (1901). "Über Toxine und Antitoxine." *Therapie der Gegenwart*: 196.

Ehrlich, P. (1904). Vorwort. *Gesammelte Abhandlungen zur Immunitätsforschung*. P. Ehrlich. Berlin.

Ehrlich, P. and J. Morgenroth (1900). "Ueber Hämolysine. Vierte Mittheilung." *Berliner klinische Wochenschrift* 37: 681–687.

Ehrlich, P. and J. Morgenroth (1904). Wirkung und Entstehung der aktiven Stoffe im Serum nach der Seitenkettentheorie. *Handbuch der pathogenen Mikroorganismen*. W. Kolle and A. Wassermann. Jena, Gustav Fischer Verlag. 4: 430–451.

Fischer, E. (1894). "Einfluss der Configuration auf die Wirkung der Enzyme." *Berichte der deutschen chemischen Gesellschaft* 27.

Fleck, L. (1980). Entstehung und Entwicklung einer wissenschaftlichen Tatsache. *Einführung in die Lehre vom Denkstil und Denkkollektiv*. Frankfurt a. M., Suhrkamp.

Gegenbaur, C. (1854). Zur Lehre vom Generationswechsel und der Fortpflanzung bei Medusen und Polypen. Berlin.

Goltz, D. (1986). "Der leere Uterus. Zum Einfluss von Harveys De generatione animalium auf die Lehren von der Konzeption." *Medizinhistorisches Journal* 21: 242–268.

Hartsoeker, N. (1678). "Extrait d'une lettre de M. Nicolas Hartsoeker écrite à l'Auteur du Journal touchant la maniere d faire les nouveaux Microscopes […]." *Journal des Scavans pour l'année LXXVIII*: 355–356.

Hartsoeker, N. (1694). Essay de Dioptrique. Paris, Jean Anisson.

Harvey, W. (1651). Exercitationes de generatione animalium. Amsterdam, Elzevir.

Heymann, B. (1928). "Zur Geschichte der Seitenkettentheorie Paul Ehrlichs." *Klinische Wochenschrift* 7: 1257–1260, 1305–1309.

Huber, L. (2009). Operationalisierung – Standardisierung – Normalisierung. Die Produktion und Visualisierung von Daten in der kognitiven Neurowissenschaft. Erkenntnis und Kritik. D. Dumbadze. Bielfeld, *Zeitgenössische Positionen*: 167–192.

Huyghens, C. (1899). Oeuvres Complètes Publiées par la Société Hollandaise des Sciences, T. 8, Correspondance 1676–1684, Den Haag, Martinus Nijhoff, No. 2117: 58–61.

Joblot, L. (1718). Descriptions et usages de plusieurs nouveaux microscopes, tant simples que composez. Paris, Jacques Collombat.

Kaestner, A. (1969). Wirbellose. *Lehrbuch der Speziellen Zoologie*. Stuttgart, Gustav Fischer, Bd. 1: 774

Kerckring, T. (1729). Opera omnia anatomica; continentia spicilegium anatomicum ostogeniam foetuum [...]. Leiden, Theodor Haak und Samuel Luchthaus.

Kowalewski, A. (1986). Die Haupteigenschaften der Philosophie des Als Ob. Die Philosophie des Als Ob und das Leben. *Festschrift zu Hans Vaihingers 80. Geburtstag. A. Seidel. Neudruck der Ausgabe Berlin 1932*, Aalen, Scientia: 227–235.

Krämer, S. (2009). Bild, Schrift, Zahl. München, Fink.

Leeuwenhoek, A. v. (1678). "Observationes [...] de Natis e semine genitali Animalculis." *Philosophical Transactions of the Royal Society of London* 142: 1040–1046 (Taf. 1013).

Leeuwenhoek, A. v. (1719). Epistola 116 [1699]. Data Ad Regiam Societatem Londinensem. In: Leeuwenhoek, A. van, *Epistolae ad Societatem Regiam Anglicam et alios illustres viros Seu Continuatio mirandorum Arcanorum Naturae detectorum* [...]. A. v. Leeuwenhoek. Leiden, Langerak: 82–94.

Lynch, M. (2006). The production of scientific images: vision and re-vision in the history, philosophy, and sociology of science. Visual cultures of science: rethinking representational practices in knowledge building and science communication. L. Pauwels. Lebanon, NH, *Dartmouth College Press*: 26–40.

Murphy, K.; Travers, P.:, Walport, M. 2009. Janeway Immunologie. 7. Aufl., Heidelberg, *Spectrum*, Akademischer Verlag

Prévost, J. L. and J. A. Dumas (1821–1822). "Sur les Animalcules spermatiques de divers Animaux." *Mémoires de la Société de Physique et d'Histoire Naturelle de Genève 1* (1): 180–207.

Redi, F. (1684). Osservazioni intorno agli animali viventi che si trovano negli animali viventi. Florenz, Piero Matini: Taf. 23, Fig. 1a,b.

Schatiloff, P. (1908). Die Ehrlichsche Seitenkettentheorie. Erläutert und bildlich dargestellt. Mit sechs Tafeln. Jena, Verlag Gustav Fischer.

Schinzel, B. (2006). Wie Erkennbarkeit und visuelle Evidenz für medizintechnische Bildgebung naturwissenschaftliche Objektivität unterminieren. Bild und Einbildungskraft. B. Hüppauf and C. Wulf. München: 354– 370.

Schurig, M. (1720). Spermatologia Historico-Medica. Seminis humani consideratio physico-medico-legalis [...]. Frankfurt a. M., Johann Beck.

Silverstein, A. M. (1989). A History of Immunology. San Diego, *Academic Press*.

Silverstein, A. M. (2002). Paul Ehrlich's receptor immunology, the magnificent obsession. San Diego, *Academic Press*.

Vaihinger, H. (1911). Die Philosophie des Als Ob. System der theoretischen, praktischen und religiösen Fiktionen der Menschheit auf Grund eines idealistischen Positivismus. Mit einem Anhang über Kant und Nietzsche. Berlin, Reuther und Reichardt

Valentin, G. (1837). "Über die Spermatozoen der Bären." *Nova Acta Physico-Medica Academiae Caesareae Leopoldino-Carolinae Naturae Curiosorum* 21: 239–244.

Vallisneri, A. (1721). Istoria della generazione dell'uomo e degli animali, se sia da'vermicelli spermatici, o dalle uova. Venedig, G. G. Hertz

RADIOLOGY, PHILOSOPHY, AND ONTOLOGY

James A. Overton and Cesare Romagnoli

ABSTRACT

Biomedical ontologies are systems of terminology that both human beings and computers can understand. They arise at the intersection of philosophy and modern information technology. As the scale, scope, and pace of medical science continue to increase, ontologies can help us to think and communicate more clearly. In this paper we describe domain ontologies, explain how they are built, and argue that radiologists can benefit greatly from their use.

1 INTRODUCTION

Radiology is central to the network of modern medical specialties. From general practitioners and specialists requesting tests, to pathologists checking biopsies, to surgeons and oncologists selecting targets, the radiologist must communicate clearly and effectively with his colleagues. The radiologist is the 'eyes' of the medical team inside the body. But how the radiologist sees though an MRI or ultrasound is nothing like how we see with our eyes, and medical images require very careful interpretation. In addition to the inherent difficulty of reading medical images, there are important practical difficulties of communicating clearly and effectively across language barriers and using specialized medical jargon. The stakes are high, since miscommunication is potentially fatal.

Radiology is a relatively new field, driven by rapid innovation in imaging modalities and information technology. Philosophy, on the other hand, is an ancient field, with roots that extend (in the Western tradition) to fifth century BCE Greece. Philosophers continue to consider perennial questions, many of which Socrates himself asked. But philosophy has not stood still these 2500 years. Contemporary philosophy is engaged with modern science and medicine and the new challenges they present.

In this paper we consider some of the ways in which contemporary philosophy can benefit modern radiology, and vice versa. Our main focus will be domain ontologies: carefully designed systems of terminology that can help radiologist conceptualize their work more precisely and communicate more clearly.

We begin by describing some of the challenges facing modern biomedicine in general and radiology in particular – challenges that domain ontologies can help solve. Domain ontologies developed at the intersection of two traditions: a venerable branch of philosophy and the modern field of artificial intelligence research. We then show how a domain ontology is built, and give examples of ontologies in bio-medicine. As we will explain, there remains work to be done to develop a domain ontology for radiology. Finally, we argue that ontologies are the best foundation on which to build next-generation structured reporting tools for radiology.

2 PROBLEMS IN MODERN RADIOLOGY

Modern science and medicine are rapidly increasing in scope, scale, and pace. Domain ontologies can help with three broad challenges which these changes bring: worldwide scope, massive scale, and electronic mediation.

Modern medicine operates on a global scale. New techniques and technologies are shared in international journals and developed by multinational companies. International exchanges are common, and patients move all over the world. Doctors and scientist speak different languages, but increasingly need to communicate across those language barriers. English is, in many ways, the de facto international language of science and medicine, but each field has its own specialized jargon. The solution to this problem is to establish a lingua franca, a standardized core of terminology that will be understood by anyone in the field. Sometimes this will require changing local practice to match the global standard.

The second challenge is the sheer amount of information that must be communicated. Radiologists now handle cases with hundreds of images, stored in massive electronic picture archiving and communications systems (PACS). These systems make new kinds of workflows possible, but they also constrain what can be done, and which systems can communicate with which other systems. In biomedical science more generally, scientists are dealing with larger and larger databases, which require specialized tools and knowledge to use effectively. We have to be careful to build systems that implement our best practices, rather than adapting our practices to whatever tool is easiest to build.

The third challenge is that communication is largely electronic, rather than personal and face-to-face. Human beings are surprisingly good at figuring out what other humans beings mean to say, especially when given the rich context of a face-to-face conversation. However we increasingly rely on machine-mediated communication, where context is impoverished. A fragment of data might have been dictated by one person, transcribed by another, selected by a text-mining program, retrieved by a database query, and read by another person years later and miles away. When the context is lost, small inconsistencies can easily multiply and lead to dangerous misinterpretation.

Domain ontologies are a step toward solving these three problems. Domain ontologies standardize the specialized terminology within a given field. Each domain ontology is limited to its domain, but they link together in an interoperable network. And domain ontologies are designed to be useful both to human beings and to computers. They are a partial but valuable solution to the challenges of biomedicine with worldwide scope, massive scale, and mediated by information technology.

3 TWO ROADS TO ONTOLOGY

The techniques for building domain ontologies arose from the intersection of two traditions. The first is a philosophical tradition stretching through biology and back to Aristotle. The second includes half a century of research into adapting human knowledge to computer applications.

3.1 Aristotle

The word 'ontology' comes from the Greek words 'ontos', for being, and 'logos', for study or science. 'The study of being' has its roots in pre-Socratic philosophy, where one of the central questions was how to understand the common nature behind the world's diversity. Several pre-Socratic philosophers proposed a single organizing principle. Heraclitus (5th century BCE) thought of the world as a process of continual change, and he is famous for saying that one cannot step into the same river twice. Parmenides (early 5th century BCE) conceived of all being as one, and essentially unchanging. Others understood all things as composed of combinations of the four elements, earth, water, air, and fire, while Leucippus (5th century BCE) and Democritus (c.460–c.370 BCE) conceived of matter as atoms in the void.

Aristotle (384–322 BCE) was a keen observer of nature, and built a broad and systematic account of what he saw. His many works include discussions of physics, metaphysics, biology, politics, art, and logic. In the *Categories* Aristotle developed a theory of definitions with which to build systematic classification systems. To define a species, we must give its genus and differentia, i. e. the broader category to which it belongs and the properties that distinguish it within that category. (The terms 'species' and 'genus' are meant generally, not in their specific biological senses.) Species are then further subdivided into finer categories. For example, Porphyry of Tyre (AD 234–c.305) applied Aristotle's method to create the Porphyrian tree, which he used to classify all substances (see Figure 1).

Aristotle's method of classification has been applied to biology, past and present. The great taxonomist Linnaeus (1707–1778) used this approach to develop his tree of life, the predecessor of modern taxonomy and cladistics. Genus-differen-

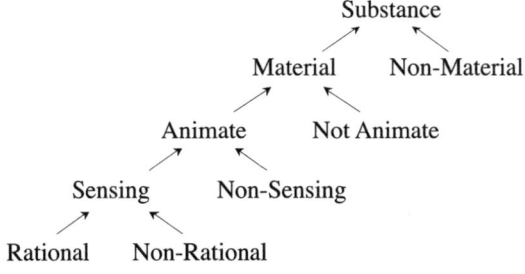

Figure 1: The Prophyrian Tree

tia definitions and Aristotle's method of division are so widely used in science and everyday life that they may seem trivial, but it is all to easy to make serious errors when designing classification systems.

3.2 Artificial Intelligence

In the summer of 1956 John McCarthy (1927–) organized the Dartmouth Summer Research Conference on Artificial Intelligence, a month-long brainstorming session that gave birth to the field of artificial intelligence research. In the decades since, AI research has had a wide influence on generations of computer scientists and computer technologies.

One branch of AI research, which came into its own in the 1970s, is called 'knowledge representation' (KR). KR researchers develop tools for formalizing knowledge in particular domains, and representing it such that computers can search and manipulate that knowledge. Although machine reasoning is very fragile, machines can follow long chains of inference across massive databases, without getting lost in the details.

KR researchers adopted the term 'ontology' from philosophy. In their usage, an ontology is a system of fundamental concepts that make reasoning about a domain of knowledge possible. A computer system may have access to a large store of facts about the world, but the ontology is the system of basic classifications that organizes those facts.

In the past decade, Sir Timothy Berners-Lee and the World Wide Web Consortium (W3C) have been pushing for widespread adoption of semantic web technologies. The semantic web builds on results and techniques from KR research, but applies them to the massive scale of the Internet. Semantic web technologies allow us to build specialized languages, to mark-up our data using those languages, and to translate between those languages. The technical details are not important here. Instead we are interested in the systems of terminology that make classification and translation possible: domain ontologies.

Domain ontologies show how techniques that date back to Aristotle can find new applications in modern information technology. Although the technology is new, what is required to use it well is careful thinking about how we should understand and classify the world.

4 BUILDING AN ONTOLOGY

To build a good domain ontology we must begin with a clearly defined domain (Arp et al. 2008). The best ontologies are tightly constrained, but also designed to interoperate with ontologies from other domains. This is one of the strengths of the Open Biomedical Ontologies project, which we discuss below. In this section we use an example drawn from the Foundational Model of Anatomy (FMA). The domain of the FMA is human anatomy: the structural organization of the human body.[1] Terms that describe diseases of the anatomy, or surgical procedures on human beings, or the anatomy of other species not shared by humans, are all excluded from the FMA. But other ontologies such as the Human Disease Ontology can refer to the FMA without having to duplicate their efforts.

Once the domain is specified, there are three steps to building a domain ontology. First, the terms must be collected and defined. Second, they must be organized into a hierarchy using a single well-defined relation. Third, additional links between terms are added to transform the hierarchy into a network. The first step creates a lexicon of terms, the second a taxonomy, and the third a domain ontology.

4.1 Lexicon

A lexicon is a list of terms and definitions. The terms will refer to universals within the domain. Universals are abstract and general things such as 'tree', 'heart', 'cell', in contrast with particular things such as the tree called 'Kiidk'yaas' that was felled on January 22, 1997, or the heart of Abraham Lincoln, or the first cell of a given stem cell line. Universals are abstract entities that are instantiated by particular entities. Universals have no location in time or space, while particulars exist at given times and places. The goal of a domain ontology is to organize the universals for a domain, give them clear definitions, and specify the relationships between them. The definitions in a lexicon should be given in Aristotelean genus-differentia form, especially if the 'is a' relation is to be used in the next step.

Figure 2 lists some terms from the FMA, denoting universals in the domain of human anatomy.

• Anatomical Space	• Anatomical Structure	• Pleural Sac
• Organ Cavity	• Organ	• Parietal Pleura
• Organ Cavity Subdivision	• Organ Part	• Mediastinal Pleura
• Serous Sac Cavity	• Serous Sac	• Pleura (Wall of Sac)
• Serous Sac Cavity Subdivision	• Organ Component	
• Pleural Cavity	• Organ Subdivision	• Visceral Pleura
• Interlobar Recess	• Tissue	• Mesothelium of Pleura

Figure 2: A list of some terms in the Foundational Model of Anatomy

4.2 Taxonomy

A taxonomy takes the terms from a lexicon and organizes them into a hierarchy. Terms are connected together using a single well-defined relation. Most taxonomies use the 'is a' relation, which relates a sub-type to its parent type (i. e. species to ge-

---

1   http://sig.biostr.washington.edu/projects/fm/AboutFM.html

nus). Some hierarchies may instead use the 'part of' relation to express containment of a sub-part inside a larger part.

Once the terms are organized into a hierarchy, it is possible to do some basic reasoning over the structure. For example, a computer can use the hierarchy to include the terms 'serous sac' and 'pleural sac' in a database search for instances of 'organ'. Figure 3 shows the 'is a' taxonomy for part of the FMA.

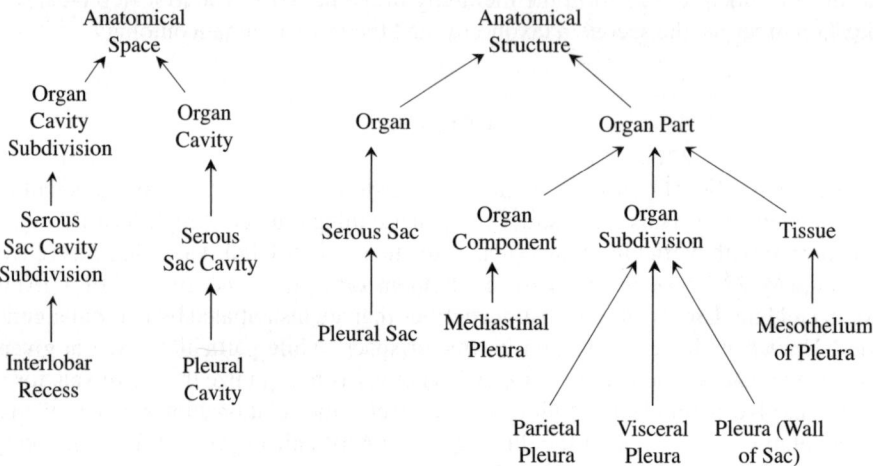

Figure 3: Some terms from the Foundational Model of Anatomy,
with arrows showing 'is a' relationships.

4.3 Domain Ontology

Finally, a domain ontology enriches the taxonomy by adding more well-defined relations connecting terms. Instead of a tree-structure, the result is a network of connections that supports more complex reasoning along the various links.

Figure 4 shows part of the FMA with both 'is a' and 'part of' relations.

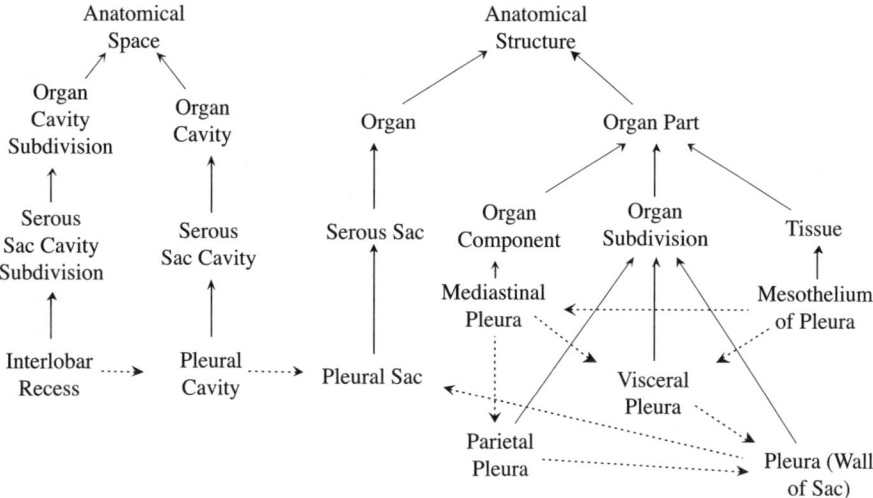

Figure 4: Some terms from the Foundational Model of Anatomy,
with solid arrows showing 'is a' relationships and dotted arrows showing 'part of' relationships.

5 BIOMEDICAL ONTOLOGIES

Ontologies are used for a wide variety of purposes, ranging from library science to military intelligence analysis. Here we are interested in ontologies for biomedicine.

5.1 SNOMED CT

Systematized Nomenclature of Medicine – Clinical Terms[2] started in 1965 under the name Systematized Nomenclature of Pathology (SNOP), grew to become SNOMED, then SNOMED RT (Reference Terminology), and then merged with the England and Wales National Health Service's Clinical Terms to become SNOMED CT. Its coverage of other medical fields has grown quickly in the last decade to be quite comprehensive. It is now the largest systematic collection of biomedical terms, including more than 311 000 concepts, and 800 000 definitions and synonyms with 1 360 000 links between them. The concepts are organized into hierarchies such as 'clinical finding/disorder', 'body structure', 'organism', 'event', etc.

SNOMED CT is becoming a widely accepted standard because of its broad coverage of terms. But it has been criticized for errors of classification (Ceusters et al. 2004), and linguistic, structural, and ontological problems (Ceusters et al. 2003; Bodenreider et al. 2007).

2   http://www.ihtsdo.org/snomed-ct/

5.2 RadLex

The Radiology Lexicon[3] was developed by the Radiology Society of North America (RSNA) to organize educational resources. Because it was not originally designed using best principles of ontology development, there have been many problems with RadLex as an ontology. In previous versions, under its top-level element 'RadLex term' there were entries for 'treatment', 'imaging observation', 'anatomic entity', 'teaching attribute', and 'image quality', among others. This demonstrates a use/mention confusion. While it is true that the phrase 'anatomic entity' is a RadLex term, it is not true that anatomical entities in the world like livers, hearts, and lungs are RadLex terms – words were being confused with their referents. RadLex also duplicates terms from other more comprehensive ontologies such as the Foundational Model of Anatomy (FMA), but there have been efforts to integrate RadLex with FMA (Mejino et al. 2008).

5.3 Open Biomedical Ontologies

The Open Biomedical Ontologies Consortium[4] brings together a number of domain ontology projects under a set of shared best practices (Smith et al. 2007). OBO Foundry ontologies have permissive licenses, use open source development tools, and share a human-readable file format. They are designed to have a good division of labour, so that a given universal is only defined in one ontology and other ontologies can link to that definition. To support interoperability, every term of every OBO ontology has a unique identifier. And all OBO Foundry ontologies share a common Basic Formal Ontology, described below. As of November 2011 there are eight OBO Foundry ontologies which implement all the best practices, and dozens of candidate ontologies that are working towards meeting all the requirements.

Here we describe some of the OBO Foundry and candidate ontologies of particular interest to radiologists.

Foundational Model of Anatomy (FMA)
The FMA includes more than 70 000 anatomical terms.[5] Its domain is human anatomy, from gross anatomy to cellular structures.

Gene Ontology (GO)
The Gene Ontology is actually three ontologies covering closely related domains: biological processes, cellular components, and molecular functions.[6] Many of the best practices of the OBO consortium were developed from the Gene Ontology project.

---

3   http://www.rsna.org/radlex/
4   http://obofoundry.org
5   http://sig.biostr.washington.edu/projects/fm/
6   http://www.geneontology.org/

Human Disease Ontology (DOID)
The Human Disease Ontology includes diseases such as cancers, infections, and mental illness.[7] In general its structure parallels the Foundational Model of Anatomy, and it includes many terms from SNOMED CT and other medical terminology systems.

Ontology for Biomedical Investigations (OBI)
OBI does not describe a scientific domain, but rather the tools, procedures, and techniques by which medicine and science are conducted. These range from computer files to investigator roles to biological specimens.[8]

Phenotype Quality (PATO)
PATO was originally designed to describe the phenotypes of organisms such as fruit flies, but has evolved to include a wide range of qualitative terms, including sizes, shapes, colours, textures, and units of measurement.[9]

While each domain ontology focuses on its own specific domain, a formal ontology is designed to be general. Like the Porphyrian tree, the Basic Formal Ontology[10] makes fundamental classifications of things. Figure 5 shows a fragment of the BFO. Some of its terms correspond to standard terms in philosophy: independent continuants are substances, dependent continuants are properties of substances, and processual entities are events. Sharing the same fundamental classifications facilitates interoperability among all the OBO ontologies.

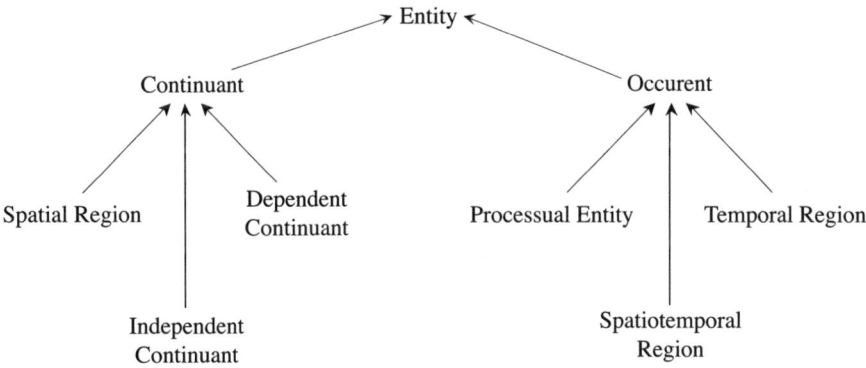

Figure 5: A fragment of the Basic Formal Ontology.

7   http://diseaseontology.sourceforge.net/
8   http://purl.obofoundry.org/obo/obi
9   http://www.bioontology.org/wiki/index.php/PATO:Main_Page
10 http://www.ifomis.org/bfo

6 ONTOLOGIES FOR RADIOLOGY

RadLex and SNOMED CT include a number of the terms that radiologists use every day in their reports and conversations. Unfortunately, many of these terms are not yet included in OBO ontologies (Overton et al. 2011). For example, OBO does not yet include any ontologies with terms for medical imaging modalities. Here is an example of some of the terms that are required in radiology:

– Magnetic Resonance Imaging (MRI) Image
  • T1 Weighted MRI Image
    ▪ MRI Image without Contrast
    ▪ MRI Image with Contrast
  • T2 Weighted MRI Image
  • Proton Density Weighted MRI Image
– Ultrasound (US) Image
– X-Ray Image
– Nuclear Medicine Image

Also required are terms for describing the radiological qualities of the observations made:

– intensity (MRI)
– echogenicity (ultrasound)
– transparency (X-Ray)
– density (CT)

And there must be terms to specify the ways in which these qualities contrast with nearby features or change over time.

– nearby tissue
– change in time
– change with contrast enhancement
– change with sequence type

The natural home for many of these terms is OBI. One of the best features of the OBO approach to ontologies is its openness, and once these terms are properly listed, defined, and related they can be proposed for inclusion into OBI.

Although terms for imaging modalities are missing, OBO contains many other needed terms. The size, location, and many of the qualitative characteristics of the features in an image can be described using PATO. The anatomy itself can be described using the FMA, and diseases of the anatomy with the Human Disease Ontology. With the addition of the radiology-specific terms just discussed, all the pieces will be in place for the use of ontologies across a wide range of communication in radiology.

7 ONTOLOGIES AND REPORTING

This paper began with a discussion of the problems of communication that radiologists face. Perhaps the most important way in which radiologists communicate with their colleagues in other disciplines is through medical reports. When a general practitioner or specialist requests a test, the radiologist returns the results in the form of a written report. Today these reports are usually text entries in a database.

If the terminology used in reports is clearly defined, communication becomes easier. And if a radiologist is trained using high-quality ontologies, not only his communication but also his thinking will be more clear. As we have discussed elsewhere (Romagnoli et al. 2010), it is valuable to distinguish between the marks we see in medical images and the interpretations we give to those marks. The French neuroradiologist Auguste Wackenheim distinguished between the sign and the signified, where the former is the mark as it appears to us, and the latter is the meaning we attach to the mark (Wackenheim 1985). The sign could be a small region in a CT scan that is darker than its surroundings. We can attach successive layers of significance to this sign. We say it is a hypodense lesion in the patient's body. It may be a cystic lesion, or a cystic tumour, or a serous adenoma. At each of these steps we are interpreting more from the image, and more likely to be making some mistake in our interpretation.

The crucial point is that we should be clear about the degree of interpretation we are making. This distinction is supported by dividing the report into sections, such as 'clinical information', 'technique of examination', 'description of findings', and 'conclusions'. Clarity will be further improved when the different sections use terms from different ontologies: 'small' and 'dark' belong to PATO; 'hypodense' should belong to a radiology ontology; 'adenoma' belongs to the Human Disease Ontology.

Another potential way to improve reporting is to use structured reports. Rather than typing or dictating a plain-text report, a radiologist creates a structured report by interacting with a computer program, clicking checkboxes and filling in input fields. He must complete all the required fields, ensuring that important information is not left out. The hierarchical and carefully coded data from a structured report should be consistent, complete, and use well-defined ontology terms. It will be much easier to search and to analyze than a plain-text report. Better reporting data means better quality assurance, easier meta-analysis, and better follow-up for patients. The main problem with structured reports is that they are much more constraining than free-form plain-text reports, and so the challenge is to design reporting tools that have enough breadth and flexibility.

There have been some recent studies on structured reporting in radiology, that have not shown clear benefits (Johnson 2002; Johnson et al. 2009; Langlotz 2009). Nevertheless, the RSNA has a Radiology Reporting Initiative to develop structured reporting templates.[11] We believe that the key to good structured reports is good conceptual foundations, which means using high-quality domain ontologies.

8 CONCLUSION

It takes years of training to read medical images well. Radiologists are challenged daily to communicate clearly and effectively about what they see. These challenges are increasing as modern medicine increases in scale, scope, and pace.

Domain ontologies are a step toward meeting these challenges. They define and systematize terminology in a way that human beings and computers can both understand. The Open Biomedical Ontologies Consortium is leading the way in best practices for ontology development and use, because they have recognized both the technical and the philosophical problems involved. We have come a long way since Aristotle, but more than ever before we need to think clearly about how we understand the world and how we communicate that understanding.

ACKNOWLEDGEMENTS

This research has been supported by grants from the Department of Medical Imaging at the London Health Sciences Centre and from the Rotman Institute of Philosophy at the University of Western Ontario, and by graduate student funding from the Social Sciences and Humanities Research Council of Canada.

REFERENCES

Arp, R., Romagnoli, C., Chhem, R.K., & Overton, J.A. (2008) 'Radiological and Biomedical Knowledge Integration: The Ontological Way', in R.K. Chhem, K.M. Hibbert, & T.V. Deven (eds.), Radiology Education: The Scholarship of Teaching and Learning (Heidelberg: Springer): 87–104.

Bodenreider, O., Smith, B., Kumar, A., & Burgun, A. (2007) 'Investigating subsumption in SNOMED CT: An exploration into large description logic-based biomedical terminologies', Artificial intelligence in medicine 39(3): 183–195.

Ceusters, W., Smith, B., & Flanagan, J. (2003). 'Ontology and Medical Terminology: Why Description Logics Are Not Enough', in Towards an Electronic Patient Record (Boston, MA: Medical Records Institute).

Ceusters, W., Smith, B., Kumar, A., & Dhaen, C. (2004) 'Mistakes in Medical Ontologies: Where Do They Come From and How Can They Be Detected?', Studies in Health Technology and Informatics 102: 145–164.

Johnson, A.J. (2002) 'Radiology Report Quality: A Cohort Study of Point-and-Click Structured Reporting versus Conventional Dictation', Academic Radiology 9(9): 1056–1061.

---

11   http://reportingwiki.rsna.org

Johnson, A. J., Chen, M. Y., Swan, J. S., Applegate, K. E., & Littenberg, B. (2009) 'Cohort Study of Structured Reporting Compared with Conventional Dictation', Radiology 253(1): 74–80.

Langlotz, C. P. (2009) 'Structured Radiology Reporting: Are We There Yet?', Radiology 253(1): 23–25.

Mejino, J. L., Rubin, D. L., & Brinkley, J. F. (2008) 'FMA-RadLex: An Application Ontology of Radiological Anatomy derived from the Foundational Model of Anatomy Reference Ontology', in American Medical Informatics Association 2008 Symposium Proceedings: 465–469.

Overton, J. A., Romagnoli, C., & Chhem, R. K. (2011) 'Open biomedical ontologies applied to prostate cancer', Applied Ontology, 6(1): 35–51.

Romagnoli, C., Overton, J. A., & Chhem, R. K. (2010) 'Philosophy in Radiology: The Ontological Challenge', in T. V. Deven, K. M. Hibbert, & R. K. Chhem (eds.), The Practice of Radiology Education (New York: Springer): 239–248.

Smith, B., Ashburner, M., Rosse, C., Bard, J., Bug, W., Ceusters, W., Goldberg, L. J., Eilbeck, K., Ireland, A., Mungall, C. J., the OBI Consortium, Leontis, N., Rocca-Serra, P., Ruttenberg, A., Sansone, S.-A., Scheuermann, R. H., Shah, N., Whetzel, P. L., & Lewis, S. (2007) 'The OBO Foundry: Coordinated evolution of ontologies to support biomedical data integration', Nature biotechnology: 25(11): 1251–1255.

Wackenheim, A. (1985) 'Cervico-Occipital Joint (RX, CT): 158 Radiological Exercises for Students and Practitioners' (Berlin: Springer-Verlag).

SCIENTIFIC IMAGES FROM FUNCTIONAL BRAIN IMAGING IN CONTEMPORARY NEUROSCIENCE – COMPLEX AND PROBLEMATIC PROCESSING PROCEDURES

Kirsten Brukamp

REFLECTING ON BRAIN IMAGES IN NEUROSCIENCE

When can images of the brain be informative about cognitive processes? What does the scientific study of neuronal activity reveal about the mind, which remains an invisible, imagined, and elusive entity? Can the concept of consciousness be captured in scientific images? Although the scope of these questions is too wide to allow a short answer, a systematic assessment of brain images offers insights into the potential propensities towards error propagation due to the highly sophisticated constructedness of these images.

Contemporary cognitive neuroscience generates highly complex images of the brain in order to draw conclusions about brain function and the interplay between various cognitive capabilities. Frequently, impressive results are presented as graphical depictions of processed brain images in the scientific literature and the popular press alike. Nevertheless, criticism from within the scientific field of the cognitive neuroscience community itself has challenged the statistical validity of some data (compare the section "Cognitive neuroscience: achievements and distractions"). Therefore, a meticulous examination of the image processing steps is required to understand the layers of image construction (compare the section "Brain images as highly processed technological products"). In this way, flawed analysis steps can be connected with the corresponding features in image representations. Modern neuroscience aims at revealing the experiment participant as a true subject and thereby strengthens a subject-oriented approach in the natural sciences (compare the section "Beginnings of a neuroscience image theory").

COGNITIVE NEUROSCIENCE: ACHIEVEMENTS AND DISTRACTIONS

Contemporary functional neuroimaging of the brain assesses higher cognitive functions in humans. This scientific aim falls into the domains of cognitive neuroscience and psychology, which investigate cognitive functions such as perception, action, emotion, decision-making, thought, and consciousness.

Functional neuroimaging, particularly functional magnetic resonance imaging (fMRI), has greatly propelled cognitive research forward. fMRI research produces images that are widely distributed in neuroscience and the public press. This phenomenon does not necessarily apply to other methods in brain research, such as electroencephalography (EEG) and magnetoencephalography (MEG), which are typically not associated with intuitively impressive images. Diffusion tensor imaging (DTI), which has not gained wide-spread lay recognition yet, produces remarkably colorful images of structural connectivity; nevertheless, DTI is not a functional method and therefore unfit for the study of cognitive psychological processes proper. Positron emission tomography (PET) is another visual technology, which is rarely used for functional studies, but instead for molecular and neuroreceptor imaging.

Either these visual techniques work primarily with images, or their data can conveniently be represented visually. Thereby, they are in contrast to the analysis of brain activity by electrophysiology in animals. Compared to other methods of brain imaging, fMRI is non-invasive and well tolerated with negligible side effects. Nowadays, structural connectivity in the intact brain can best be studied with DTI, whereas fMRI permits conclusions about functional connectivity in the living brain, enabling implications for effective connectivity.

In face of the ambitious research program of cognitive neuroscience, it is not surprising that the intense research environment in functional neuroimaging has led to the identification of problematic issues in functional neuroimaging related to fMRI data, images, and statistics. In recent years, there has been strong criticism regarding some types of statistical analysis that are employed in functional MRI. This criticism has come from the community itself: A subgroup of researchers began to look at methods of statistical analysis from a highly critical perspective. These researchers have suggested that some effects may be inflated because of a tendency to obtain false positive results due to a wrong application of statistics.

Vul et al. (2009) examined the statistical calculations upon which the neuroscientific reports of fMRI research are based.[1] In more than half of the cases, they identified the use of non-independent analysis: First, correlations for individual voxels were computed, and then, means for selected significant voxels were reported. This procedure inflates the statistical result considerably because the individual voxels are pooled: A report based on the combination is in principle more impressive than the individual ones. Under these conditions, high correlation coefficients, sometimes in excess of 0.8 or even 0.95, are obtained between brain activity and social and emotional measures, such as psychological scales. Vul et al. (2009) were able to show that the correlations were indeed higher for the studies that performed the erroneous statistics than for studies that did not.

Vul et al. (2009) suspect that this type of non-independence error is not limited to fMRI research in the field of social neuroscience – which they define as the study of emotion, personality, and social cognition –, but occurs in all areas of neuroscience that utilize fMRI. Does this suspicion undermine the validity of cognitive psychology at large? It certainly does not falsify fMRI results qualitatively. After all, numerous studies have applied the statistical tests correctly, and scientists typi-

---

1   Prior to publication, this study by Vul et al. (2009) was referred to by the former title "Voodoo correlations in social neuroscience". The study elicited considerable interest, in part due to its provocative heading.

cally look for several reports that go in the same direction and strengthen mutual conclusions. On the other hand, publication bias already leads to an inflation of statistical values in the literature anyway because only significant results are typically published and reports on weak or non-existent associations rarely appear in scientific journals.

Bennett, a postdoctoral researcher in psychology at the University of California in Santa Barbara, was capable of demonstrating the "fishy" origin of some fMRI data in a highly memorable way (Bennett et al. 2009): He placed a dead salmon inside an MRI scanner, and he subjected the lifeless fish to the same emotional and social tasks that are normally used for humans – explicitly, to determine emotions in pictures of humans. Although the animal did not exhibit any brain activity at all, the statistical analysis without correction for multiple comparisons yielded a significant result for a cluster of voxels in the brain. This was not the case when a correction for multiple comparisons was applied, specifically a control for the false discovery rate (FDR) and the family-wise error rate (FWER). The false-positive effect can be explained, at least in part, by the tendency of voxels with higher mean intensity to possess higher standard deviations and to form spatial clusters.

The study by Bennett et al. (2009) elicited considerable scientific and popular attention, partly because of the unconventional approach to tackle the problem, partly because of the visualization that it uses, and partly because of its implications. Perhaps it is particularly efficient to criticize an image with another image. Palpable positive effects of the study, which are already being seen, include a stricter emphasis on correction for multiple comparisons in peer review.

The fact that the criticism about statistical measures arose from within the scientific community indicates that its purpose lies in furthering the progress in the field – even the critics themselves offer routes to solutions. One suggestion is the use of a principled approach, with principled corrections[2] (Bennett et al. 2009), which can be achieved by the above-mentioned correction for multiple comparisons by controls for the false discovery rate (FDR) and the family-wise error rate (FWER).

General recommendations on resolving the problematic issues include the strategies to foster awareness of the critical points, develop standardized approaches, share algorithms and computational tools for peer review, and teach statistics to students. It is important to clearly distinguish experimental course and low-level data interpretation from theory and high-level interpretation. For example, even MRI images can be regarded as low-level data on the basis of the advanced stage that the technology has reached, whereas complex statistics can be considered a higher-level interpretation. As always, efficient peer review can detect pitfalls and refer discrepancies back to those who are most familiar with the studies – the experimenters.

---

2   "By principled, we mean a correction that definitively identifies for the reader the probability or the proportion of false positives that could be expected in the reported results." (Bennett et al. 2009: 417)

BRAIN IMAGES AS HIGHLY PROCESSED TECHNOLOGICAL PRODUCTS

For an assessment of the role that images take in science, a mere look at the final image as an end result is not sufficient. The procedure by which a figure of a published scientific article is obtained proves equally important. Accordingly, the technical background and the processing steps for fMRI are summarized in the following, in part according to typical features in common fMRI analysis software packages (Ashburner et al. 2010; Goebel et al. 2008).

Regarding the technical basics, fMRI relies on the reporting of the blood-oxygenation level dependent (BOLD) signal. Thereby, it does not constitute a direct measure of neuronal activity, but rather an indirect measure of increased perfusion at the sites of intense neuronal workload. Typically, the spatial resolution is one to several cubic millimeters and the temporal resolution is one to several seconds; however, values of below one millimeter and less than 0.5 seconds have already been reached as well. The spatial resolution of fMRI is considered more valuable than its temporal one because the former is relatively high in comparison to other functional neuroimaging methods. Thus, fMRI is occasionally combined with simultaneous EEG to obtain better insights into the time dimension as well. The scope of fMRI is reflected in the increasing number of publications on studies that have utilized it over the last decades.

Before the fMRI image analysis even begins, most technical data have already been fixed during the experimental acquisition procedure: image type, magnetic field strength, numbers of rows and columns, pixel size, slice thickness, spacing between slices or gap thickness, repetition time (TR), and echo time (TE) (Goebel et al. 2008: 10–11). In addition, the experimenter's expertise has shaped an experimental protocol that needs to be fixed in the image analysis software as the stimulation protocol. Conditions also may be, but do not have to be, graphically defined via a time course plot. Conditions can only be compared after researchers account for the hemodynamic delay in the fMRI response relative to the neuronal activity. This is done by applying a hemodynamic response function (HRF), which may be a previously described pre-defined or a self-defined model function.[3] So-called preprocessing steps are meant to improve the quality of the data prior to analysis. Preprocessing options include mean intensity adjustment, slice scan time correction, 3D motion correction, spatial smoothing, and temporal filtering (Goebel et al. 2008: 21–23). The 3D motion correction step eliminates head movement artifacts, and several mathematical types of interpolation may be utilized. Six types of corrections take place, namely both three translations and three axial rotations for the three dimensions. Spatial smoothing involves the application of a Gaussian filter with the options of an absolute (millimeter) or relative (pixel) length in the space

---

3   Most analyses apply one standard HRF to the whole brain, although each brain region probably has its own HRF and HRFs are dependent on the size of the activated population (Logothetis 2008: 877). Obviously, this common procedure results in errors, and it is currently inestimable to which degree the practice undermines the validity of the data.

domain. Nevertheless, the use of spatial smoothing in preprocessing is usually considered unnecessary or even dubious because of its tendency to alter the data too much. Temporal filtering is important for the removal of drifts in signal time courses and can consider both linear and non-linear trends. A valuable option is the application of a temporal high pass filter to remove slow drift artifacts.

The spatial analysis of the functional data requires a comparison with an anatomical scan that represents morphology with a high spatial resolution in the sagittal, coronal, and transverse views. The alignment of the different image types is known as coregistration. It allows the identification of brain regions for the functional data. Moreover, a standardization in stereotactic space is feasible, e. g. in Talairach space (Talairach and Tournoux 1988), rather than just in space relative to the study data. For the Talairach transformation, reference points have to be specified, and the transformation then uses an interpolation to fit the real brain to a standard brain, so that a common reference frame may be applied to all brains examined. Locations for the brain can thereafter be reported as either system or Talairach three-dimensional coordinates.

For some analyses, it is useful to obtain surface visualizations of the head or the brain so that the head surface can be related to the brain images inside the head. Another conceivable application is the spatial coregistration of fMRI data with EEG or MEG data, when the latter are available. In addition, it may be worthwhile to view data after cortical flattening.

Cortex segmentation and reconstruction may be done for the boundaries between white and gray matter or the boundary between outer gray matter and pia mater. This procedure involves many computational steps such as smoothing, filling of ventricles, finding intensity peaks for gray and white matter, and segmenting of white matter (Goebel et al. 2008: 78 ff.). Cortex inflation then generates a surface map that allows the equal inspection of regions on gyri and in sulci. Color options include either a two-color code for convex gyri and concave sulci or gradual color scales for the degree of convexity and concavity. Cortex flattening includes cutting, unfolding, and distortion correction (Goebel et al. 2008: 85 ff.). The cortex is projected onto a two-dimensional flat plane. Statistical maps are conveniently displayed as overlays on cortex meshes.

Statistical information is usually reported alongside the image. Such data comprise the type of test, the degrees of freedom (when applicable), and the p value of the test, which indicates the significance, according to a pre-specified threshold. In addition, a correction for multiple comparisons may already be included in the software package in the format of the default threshold, the false discovery rate (FDR). Select pixels in the images are colored according to a color bar, which indicates color codes for p values. The statistical information of a certain region can preferentially be shown after selection of a region of interest (ROI). For a linear correlation map as an example of a statistical test, the time course of each pixel over all slices is correlated with the reference time course of the experimental conditions. Voxel-based morphometry (VBM) is the basis for statistical tests that compare volumes among populations of subjects. These can only be performed after spatial normalization of the brains of all subjects to a standard space.

One prominent type of statistical analysis is the analysis by fitting of a general linear model (GLM). A model is fitted to the time course of each voxel, and a statistical value is calculated that indicates the quality of the explanation for this time course. The GLM contains explanatory variables as predictors, which are assigned estimated effects on the time series, so that their relative contributions can be compared. In other words, the variation of the time course is explained as a linear combination of explanatory variables. GLM analysis includes the following steps (Ashburner et al. 2010: 61): 1. preparation of the data and construction of a design matrix, 2. estimation of GLM parameters, and 3. application of the results to the data and visualization by statistical parametric maps (SPMs) or posterior probability maps (PPMs).

The output of the GLM results can take very different, but complementary formats: 1. a depiction of the statistical information in the images by color-coding, 2. a table with statistical values for significance tests, predictor weights, and multiple correlation values, and 3. a comparative graph of the data, the model, and the residual curves for a simple visual impression of the goodness of fit.

Statistical tests also compare sets of voxels regarding patterns of activity by multivariate approaches. Another option for classifying output is by support vector machines (SVMs), which are useful as machine learning tools when the magnitude and complexity of the data do not allow easy categorization. SVMs discriminate activity patterns in new studies after training with standard data, and they predict the correct class for the test data.

In summary, generating meaningful images out of experimental functional neuroimaging data is a multi-step, complex procedure. The final end product of processing oftentimes presents morphological information and statistical analysis together. There are a number of discrepancies concerning the status of fMRI images: The images suggest simplicity, but they are highly processed. They seem objective, like spoken words and written texts, but purposeful or unintentional falsification is possible. The images suggest evidence, but they require interpretation. They seem quasi-natural, but they are construed.[4] Although the images draw the onlookers' attention because of their low-threshold visual attractiveness, they are not readily accessible to laypeople upon closer inspection.

This review demonstrates the multifarious applications of and intentions for color-coding in neuroimaging:[5] 1. Color-coding is used to convey morphological information, in order to highlight structures. 2. Color-coding can represent statisti-

---

4   "By applying the imaging tools developed for scientific purposes to objects of the everyday world, you demonstrate the constructive nature of the allegedly objective imaging technologies. [These, K. B.] works make it intuitively understandable that the world as we perceive it is the result of construction and that what we perceive is nothing but an idiosyncratic interpretation of the world." (Leidloff and Singer 2008: 234)

5   Information may be depicted in gray-scale, so that shades of black and white serve as a code, but the focus here is on hybrid fMRI data and therefore on colors. – In general, questions about the purpose and the effect of using color-coding *versus* a gradual black-and-white scale in biomedical contexts (Groß and Schäfer 2007: 277) are highly relevant to contemporary neuroimaging, but this topic cannot be addressed here.

cal information, either 2.1 absolute statistical values or 2.2 relative statistical values, i.e. differences between hemispheres or brain regions. Thereby, it is either 1. coding for space or 2. for numbers. In both cases, the non-visual representation is definitively too complex. Therefore, images are needed to represent the data, despite the critical issues discussed. There does not seem to be an alternative to the use of images for the depiction of the highly sophisticated information from neuroscience. In general, there is no alternative to the use of images in science when it is necessary to depict visual evidence and to arrange non-visual data graphically.

BEGINNINGS OF A NEUROSCIENCE IMAGE THEORY

Functional brain imaging in cognitive neuroscience is a scientific discipline that primarily relies on images for performing analyses, providing evidence, and communicating results. Therefore, the character of its images needs to become a focus of both neuroscience proper and the philosophy of neuroscience. Contemporary brain research promises to provide insight into higher cognitive capabilities, a circumstance that justifies a particular interest in and scrutiny of the related scientific procedures and products alike. The analysis of functional brain imaging requires a multitude of steps, and knowledge about its intricacies aids in identifying the components of the analytic procedure where improvement is warranted. Although functional neuroimaging utilizes a technology-intense approach in its pursuit of studying psychological topics, it will ultimately reveal and represent the human as the subject with individual traits that he already is – an aim that lies close to its heart.

REFERENCES

Ashburner, John, Gareth Barnes, Chun-Chuan Chen, Jean Daunizeau, Guillaume Flandin, Karl Friston, Stefan Kiebel, James Kilner, Vladimir Litvak, Rosalyn Moran, Will Penny, Klaas Stephan, Darren Gitelman, Rik Henson, Chloe Hutton, Volkmar Glauche, Jeremie Mattout, Christophe Phillips (2010) *SPM8 manual* (London: Wellcome Trust Centre for Neuroimaging, UCL).

Bennett, Craig M., Abigail A. Baird, Michael B. Miller, George L. Wolford (2009) *Neural correlates of interspecies perspective taking in the post-mortem Atlantic Salmon: an argument for multiple comparisons correction.* (Abstract at the 15th Annual Meeting of the Organization for Human Brain Mapping. San Francisco. Internet: prefrontal.org/files/posters/Bennett-Salmon-2009. pdf on June 30, 2010).

Bennett, Craig M., George L. Wolford, Michael B. Miller (2009) 'The principled control of false positives in neuroimaging', *SCAN* 4: 417–422.

Goebel, Rainer, Henk Jansma, Jochen Seitz, Armin Heinecke (2008) *Brain Voyager QX: getting started guide version 2.6.* (Maastricht: Brain Innovation).

Groß, Dominik, Gereon Schäfer (2007) ,Das Gehirn in bunten Bildern. Farbstrategien und Farbsemantiken in den Neurowissenschaften', in Dominik Groß, Stefanie Westermann (eds) (2007), *Vom Bild zur Erkenntnis? Visualisierungskonzepte in den Wissenschaften* (Kassel: Kassel University Press): 271–282.

Leidloff, Gabriele, Wolf Singer (2008) 'Neuroscience and contemporary art: an interview', in Bernd
    Hüppauf, Peter Weingart (eds) (2008), *Science images and popular images of the sciences*
    (New York: Routledge): 227–238.
Logothetis, Nikos K. (2008) 'What we can do and what we cannot do with fMRI', *Nature* 453(7197):
    869–878.
Vul, Edward, Christine Harris, Piotr Winkielman, Harold Pashler (2009) 'Puzzlingly high correla-
    tions in fMRI studies of emotion, personality, and social cognition', *Perspectives on Psycho-
    logical Science* 4(3): 274–290.

THE INHERITANCE, POWER AND PREDICAMENTS OF THE 'BRAIN-READING' METAPHOR[1]

Frédéric Gilbert, Lawrence Burns, Timothy M. Krahn

ABSTRACT

Purpose: With the increasing sophistication of neuroimaging technologies in medicine, new language is being sought to make sense of the findings. The aim of this paper is to explore whether the 'brain-reading' metaphor used to convey current medical or neurobiological findings imports unintended significations that do not necessarily reflect the genuine findings made by physicians and neuroscientists.

Methods: First, the paper surveys the ambiguities of the readability metaphor, drawing from the history of science and medicine, paying special attention to the sixteenth through nineteenth centuries. Next, the paper addresses more closely the issue of how metaphors may be confusing when used in medicine in general, and neuroscience in particular. The paper then explores the possible misleading effects associated with the contemporary use of the 'brain-reading' metaphor in neuroimaging research.

Results: Rather than breaking new ground, what we see in current scientific language is a persistence of both a constraining and expansive set of language practices forming a relatively continuous tradition linking current neuroimaging to past scientific investigations into the brain.

Conclusions: The use of the readability metaphor thus carries with it both positive and negative effects. Physicians and neuroscientists must resort to the use of terms already laden with predetermined meaning(s), and often burdened by tradition, at the risk of importing through these words connotations that do not tally with the sought-after objectivity of empirical science.

INTRODUCTION

Increasing medical sophistication in neuroimaging technologies has not only contributed to the accuracy of neuronal mapping and diagnosis, but has also generated numerous metaphors associated with the potential readability of the brain in the scientific literature. Indeed, a cursory internet search of the *Nature Publishing Group* archives from January 2006 to April 2009 (see table 1) reveals several academic articles utilizing the 'brain-reading' metaphor. For instance, in a recent publication, a neuroscientist affirmed that, even if much work is involved, "the possi-

---

1   A previous copy of this paper has been published with *Medicine Studies*.

Table 1: Textual evidence of how various authors write about "reading the brain", "reading the mind"

The following examples given below are the results of an internet search of journals from the *Nature Publishing Group* archives (January 2006 – April 2009). The table is meant only as a sampling of evidence of the brain/mind-reading metaphor. We have chosen *Nature Publishing Group* simply because it is one of the highest impact factor publishers in the field of science in general as well as neuroscience in particular. As such, it can be regarded as a very influential media that both reflects and shapes the relevant discourse(s) on this subject. This table is simply provided as a set of examples and is not meant to be understood as representative of the discourse of the "brain-reading" metaphor. The locutions searched include "reading the brain", "reading mind", "neural code", and "neural signature". Any occurrence of mind-reading referred to as "empathy" has not been included in this list.

Part 1: examples (not exhaustive) of metaphors referring to "brain reading"	Year of publication
– "Neurotechnologies such as brain reading" (Conti & Corbellini, 2008)	2008
– "Developments in neuroimaging (…) including the reading of brain states" (De Charms, 2008)	2008
– "possibility of directly reading aspects of a person's brain-activation state" (De Charms, 2008)	2008
– "general brain-reading device that could reconstruct a picture" (Kay et al., 2008)	2008
– "useful in reading the brain states" (De Charms, 2008)	2008
– "rtfMRI can potentially read complex brain states" (De Charms, 2008)	2008
– "applications for reading brain signals" (De Charms, 2008)	2008
– "'brain-reading' algorithms" (Op de Beeck et al., 2008)	2008
– "decode a person's conscious experience based on (…) 'brain reading'" (Haynes & Rees, 2006)	2006

Part 2: examples (not exhaustive) of metaphors referring to "mind reading"	Year of publication
– "reading out a person's thoughts does exist" (Anonymous, 2009)	2009
– "Mind-reading with a brain scan" (Smith, 2008)	2008
– "rtfMRI increases (…) our ability to 'read' mental states by decoding this information" (De Charms, 2008)	2008
– "directly reading a person's ongoing mental images" (De Charms, 2008)	2008
– "related methods, with the goal of mind reading" (De Charms, 2008)	2008
– "Such feats of rudimentary 'mind-reading'" (Owen & Coleman, 2008)	2008
– "Explicitly explores 'mind-reading' but with respect to tracking micro-saccades" (Martinez-Conde & Macknik, 2007)	2007
– "new ways of enhancing, controlling and reading the mind." (Stefansson, 2007)	2007
– "the possibility of "reading" a person's thoughts (…) with only his or her mind." (Schrock, 2007)	2007
– "the power of fMRI to read and predict human experience" (Anonymous, 2006)	2006
– "some even liken it to mind-reading" (Pearson, 2006)	2006
– "reading the private intentions of a person" (Amodio & Frith, 2006)	2006

Idiom	Number of articles
– Neural code	33
– Neural signature	11

bility of *reading* out a person's thoughts [from their brain] does exist" (Anonymous 2009). Indeed, sentences such as "reading the private intentions of a person" from the brain (Amodio & Frith 2006), or the ability to "decod[e] mental states from brain activity in humans" (Haynes & Rees 2006), or even claims to "mind-reading with a brain scan" (Smith 2008) are not uncommon uses of the 'brain-reading' metaphor (see table 1, part 1 for more examples). The common factor throughout these metaphors is the implicit assumption that it is possible to extract a special, perhaps temporarily hidden, signification from the 'neural muddle' of the brain with neuroimaging: indeed, idioms such as 'neural signature' and 'neural code' (see table 1, part 2) are now part of accepted and shared interdisciplinary terminologies which have proven to be, in effect, mutually reinforcing.

With the increasing sophistication of neuroimaging technologies in neuro-science research and medicine, new language is being sought to make sense of the findings. This paper demonstrates that the current project of understanding and ex-plaining the brain through neuroimaging that claims to make it 'readable', has sig-nificant precedents throughout the history of science in the West. It is our view that the 'brain-reading' metaphor, across its uses in science and medicine, has had and still has both a restrictive and expansive effect on our understanding of this most mysterious organ, the brain. The aim of this paper is to explore whether the 'brain-reading' metaphor used to convey current medical or neurobiological findings im-ports unintended significations that do not necessarily reflect the genuine findings made by physicians and neuroscientists.

To assess the value of the 'brain-reading metaphor' in its relevant contempo-rary application for making sense of investigations into the brain through neuroim-aging, we do well to consider what grounds it. First, the paper surveys the ambi-guities of the readability metaphor, drawing from the history of science and medi-cine, paying special attention to the sixteenth though nineteenth centuries. Next, the paper addresses more closely the issue of how metaphors may be confusing when used in medicine in general, and neuroscience in particular. The paper then explores the possible misleading effects associated with the contemporary use of the 'brain-reading' metaphor in neuroimaging research and its relevant applications. The pa-per concludes that rather than breaking new ground, what we see in current scien-tific language is a persistence of both a constraining and expansive set of language practices forming a relatively continuous tradition linking current neuroimaging to past medical and scientific investigations into the brain. The use of the readability metaphor thus carries with it both positive and negative effects.

1. HISTORICAL PRECEDENTS OF THE READING METAPHOR

1.1 Reading the universe

In general terms, reading is a complex cognitive process by which the ordered presentation of linguistic materials (e. g. printed characters, visual symbols, works of art) is decoded for the purposes of deriving and/or constructing meaning (cf. Goodman 2000). The intelligibility of any given text depends on the logic or system by means of which the signs relate to one another or refer beyond themselves. While a written text may serve as the paradigm for reading, non-linguistic and naturally occurring signs may also be read as texts in the relevant sense (Peirce 1998). The 'readability' of the universe (or 'legibility', as Blumenberg (1981) calls it in his extensive elucidation of the metaphor) carries with it connotations of a grand unveiling of a hidden truth about the natural world. It thus invokes the tradition of the *Book of Secrets* going back to the Middle Ages, if not further (cf. Eamon 1994).

The power and scope of the reading metaphor was definitively established during the Renaissance. In almost unprecedented fashion, Galileo Galilei's revolutionary discoveries in physics were predicated on the metaphor of a readable universe. In the context of his rejection of Scholastic doctrines concerning the solar system, Galileo asserted in the *Assayer* (1623) that:

> "Philosophy is written in this grand book, the universe, which stands continually open to our gaze. But the book cannot be understood unless one first learns to comprehend the language and read the letters in which it is composed. It is written in the language of mathematics, and its characters are triangles, circles, and other geometric figures without which it is humanly impossible to understand a single word of it; without these, one wanders about in a dark labyrinth." (Galileo 1957: 237–8)

The consequence of this view is that scientists would have to develop a new rationalist discourse in order to interpret the book of the universe (writ large) as well as its various component systems (as per the natural sciences).

1.2 Reading the body

The drive to make sense of our corporeal existence through science has across various epochs also propelled a view of the 'readability' of the body. In this regard, the human body is certainly not a conventional text; however, novel developments in anatomy in the sixteenth century helped to re-conceptualize the body as a text that could be read.

Thus the readability metaphor played a key role in establishing the scientific legitimacy of anatomy in the century before Galileo, albeit in much less direct fashion. The most exemplary and ground-breaking anatomical work in this regard is Andreas Vesalius' *De Humani Corporis Fabrica*, the publication of which in 1543 constituted a scathing critique of Church dogma and helped to clear the way for a new approach to anatomy and medicine. For almost a millennium and a half, the Christian Church had not strayed from the traditional model of human anatomy derived from Galen of Pergamum's animal dissections and his theory of the bodily humours (i.e., blood, phlegm, yellow bile and black bile). Although Galen was certainly a profoundly innovative and successful physician, experimental physiologist, writer and public orator in second-century Rome, his anatomy work was problematic on at least two accounts. First, Galen did not use human cadavers in his research. Instead, he dissected animals such as pigs and apes and then tried to apply his insights via analogy to human bodies. One of the most egregious examples of the errors caused by this approach was the claim that humans, like oxen, had a set of vessels called the *rete mirabile* at the base of the brain (Martensen 2004: 61). Second, even when the use of human cadavers was no longer prohibited in medieval universities, the authoritarian use of Galen's texts inhibited innovation and discovery. That is to say, anatomy instruction was hopelessly mired in tradition, particularly where the strict dichotomy between the priest's role as 'educated commentator' and the dissector's role as 'manual labourer' was concerned. Vesalius heaps much scorn on this practice in his *De Humani Corporis Fabrica* when he compares the priests to 'jackdaws' who sit in their 'high chairs' telling the illiterate surgeons below what to cut, neither party really knowing what they were doing (Vesalius 1998:lv). Vesalius' text corrected this schism by drawing attention to the intelligibility of the actual human body (rather than Galen's defective animal-based texts) and by intending his anatomy atlas to be used as a practical *aid* to dissection – to *look* inside human cadavers – rather than a substitute for first-hand experience. Early modern science thereafter sought to find what Vesalius referred to as the 'fabric' of the human body (Zwart 1998: 116). But, as Hub Zwart, notes, the 'fabric' of the human body was not thought of as "something which could be recognized immediately" (114): in other words, this fabric was not thought to be simply observable.

It should be apparent that the preceding description of Vesalius' work does not make direct reference to the reading metaphor. In contrast to the explicit use of the metaphor by Galileo, the readability metaphor nevertheless functions as a guiding principle or underlying paradigm for anatomy during the Renaissance. To see this, it is necessary to engage in a more extensive analysis of the socio-cultural context within which anatomy developed, drawing on some recent work in science and technology studies (STS). Pioneered by Thomas Kuhn and Michel Foucault in the 1960s, STS has become a rich source of insight into how scientific inquiry is socially situated or constructed (cf. Golinski 2005; Hacking 2007; Sismondo, 2010). Lorraine Daston and Peter Galison illustrate this attitude to science in their book *Objectivity* (2007) by elucidating how the content of scientific inquiry is shaped in part by the methodology or standpoint of the inquirer. This is not to say that scientific facts are arbitrary or wholly dependent on conceptual schemes. Rather (as the discussion of Foucault below will demonstrate), new configurations of social institutions (e.g., the hospital and the university) may be productive and stimulate discovery. In the case of anatomy, Catherine Waldby (2000) draws on the work of Daston and Galison, Jonathan Sawday and Bruno Latour to document the influence of technology and the reading metaphor on the science of anatomy.

Reflecting on the differences between modern computer-generated anatomical models and Renaissance anatomy atlases, Waldby notes that in each case the form of representation helps to construct the object represented (i.e., the content). In particular, the two-dimensional medium of the printed page and the mass production afforded by the printing press created new opportunities for Vesalius at the same time as they placed new constraints on the representation of the human body. Some of these constraints included the need to clearly demarcate tissues, to hide fluids, and to add colour coding (Waldby 2000: 98), but the most significant was the requirement that the body be represented spatially as a series of two-dimensional maps that could be overlaid upon one another (rather than as a volume of matter subject to putrefaction and decay).

The methodology presupposed by the anatomical atlas introduced an essential analogy between the cadaver on the dissection table and a text that was open to reading (especially since both have a spine) (Sawday 1995: 132; Martensen 2004). The atlas therefore consisted of a 'flayed' body (much like the modern CT scan slices stored in a data archive (Hutson 2005)) whose secrets were readily accessible to the reader who used the book as a map to guide the process and situate the findings of dissection (Waldby 2000: 94). As a result of this complementary relationship between the act of dissecting and the representation of that act in textual form, Waldby concludes that:

> In this sense the 'anatomical' body and the anatomical text were 'co-emergent', coming into being only in relationship to each other. Moreover, the anatomical body is produced only in the act of dis-integration, becoming fully anatomical only in the acts of surgery or anatomical dissection, that is, in the act of being anatomically 'written'. (Waldby 2000: 91–2)

The extent to which this interpretive anatomization of the body as text is a creative act (but no less objective for all that) is explored in greater detail below in the discussion of the difference between reading and seeing in the context of Foucault's STS work.

1.3 Reading the brain

After years of stagnation, anatomical research and teaching continued to develop by building on the legacy of Vesalius. This is especially true of neuro-anatomy, which demands extreme care on the part of the anatomist to preserve the fragile brain and identify its detailed structures. As Martensen has documented in *The Brain Takes Shape* (2004), the late seventeenth century was a particularly innovative time for research into brain anatomy, largely thanks to the work of Thomas Willis and his colleagues at Oxford. Following improvements at mapping the brain's physiology, the focus turned to brain function in the eighteenth century. It is at this time that the reading metaphor reasserted itself with regard to research into the brain. Specifically, the goal became to read the thoughts in the brain rather than to map the brain. The Walloon doctor Guillaume-Lambert Godart (1721–1794) discusses very explicitly the possibility of reading the brain in his 1755 treatise, *La Physique de l'Âme Humaine* (Physic of Human Soul). Godart was interested to establish the corporeal localization of the mind's abilities. He claimed that every sensation, as well as every idea, imprints a specific characteristic of the mind upon the fibres of the corpus callosum. Godart explains this cerebral 'printing' process as follows:

> [These imprints] are definite physical modifications of the acting fibre [...]. Every man's brain contains the history of his life, interior as well as exterior, spelled out in real letters, but [these letters] belong to a specific language that nature uses to address us all. Thus, an anatomist, with either very good eyes or a perfect microscope capable of seeing these letters, and with an ability to comprehend their signification, might be able to read a dead person's brain, the thoughts he or she might have had during his or her lifetime. (Godart 1755: 209–210. Translation by F. Gilbert)[2]

Godart's eighteenth-century theory explicitly suggests that a perfect seeing of the brain with "good" (presumably well-trained) eyes or vision enhancing technologies will allow the investigator to read the very essence of the brain. On Godart's view, the laws of nature work through the fibres in the same way for all people making the imprinting process on the fibres standard across different brains (Godart 1755: 359); however, the actual 'print out' of sensations as cerebral letters (by way of the rustling of fibres in the brain (Godart 1755: 174–175)) is distinct for each individual as dictated by subjective experience (Godart 1755: 359). Although Godart's use of the 'readability-of-the-brain' metaphor represented a new way of talking about the brain that had the potential to be revelatory, Godart himself held that with the state of human 'industry' (presumably, technology) at the time, there would be almost no chance that anyone could ever perfectly understand the subtle neural anatomy enough to distinguish the brains of markedly different human subjects. As he writes: "At the point where things are now, we are very far from being able to draw such distinctions; even Malpighi was unable, despite all his dexterity, to discover the difference between the brains of the great Lancisius[3], and one of the biggest idiots" (Godart 1755: 210). In the end, Godart adopted a cautious scepticism, noting that even if one were able to *see* the cerebral fibres as letters of the alphabet of the mind, this would not yet constitute knowledge of their meaning as sensible expressions of the brain-fibre language remained for him practically hermetic – no more than a theoretical postulate (Godart 1755: 210).

Nevertheless, five years later, the Parisian doctor Antoine Le Camus explained in his *Memoire on the Brain* that, with the help of his scalpel, he had searched for connections between the structure of the brain and the organization of thought. But, he noted, "I can only see a greyish mass, furrowed by smooth rays that converge into a very white mass. Unsatisfied, I therefore no longer trust my eyes only, as they are unable to let me see more organization within the Brain's substance" (Le Camus et al. 1760: 3–4). Feeling helpless, he turned to the available technological support of that epoch, the magnifying glass as well as the microscope (see Wilson 1995; Smith 2010). Even so, he met with disappointment as he was unable to find any

---

2   All subsequent English translations of Godart are provided by (first author) Frédéric Gilbert.
3   Marcello Malpighi was a 17th-century Italian doctor famous for his contributions in physiology. Lancisius was an Italian anatomist who wrote a monograph on the sympathetic nerves.

trace of the sought after neural fibres from which he had hoped to read the brain and in so doing discern its nature (Le Camus et al. 1760: 3–4).

Thus we see in the historical examples given above a belief in, or hope for, the readability of the brain as a kind of text: hence the metaphor, 'reading the brain'. But as Rabinowitz aptly notes, "a reader can only make sense of a text in the same way he or she makes sense of anything else in the world: by applying a series of strategies to simplify it – by highlighting, by making symbolic, and by otherwise patterning it" (Rabinowitz 1998: 19). Treating the brain as a readable entity in and of itself is not yet misleading, but we do well to investigate not only from whence this metaphor has come to us (as detailed above), but more generally how it, like metaphors more generally in medicine, has the capacity not only to reveal but also to conceal or distort the reported findings.

2. METAPHORS THAT SOMETIMES CONFUSE: SEEING AND READING AS METAPHORS IN MEDICINE

According to the *Oxford English Dictionary*, metaphor is defined as "a figure of speech in which a name or descriptive word or phrase is transferred to an object or action different from, but analogous to, that to which it is literally applicable" (OED 2010). Metaphors play a very important role in medicine, as in many other fields, but we do not always appreciate their implications and their potentially distorting consequences. After all, language has many metaphorical dimensions that are sometimes hidden from – or at least not explicitly apparent to – us but whose pervasiveness and guiding power help us to make sense of our experience of the world (Lakoff & Johnson 1980). In medicine, metaphors such as the 'war on disease', 'pulling the plug', and the search for a 'miracle cure' help to guide our thinking about the nature of medicine. In *Practical Reasoning in Bioethics*, James Childress presents an extensive list of medical metaphors but cautions us to be aware of the implications of using them uncritically (Childress 1997). While metaphors can illuminate aspects of phenomena that remain hidden, they can also be extremely limiting and may distort reality. In this regard, we are not always in control of our metaphors, especially when they are engrained in the way we speak and experience the world. Nevertheless, metaphors are both useful and inescapable, so we should learn how to reflect on them and use them properly (or draw attention to their misleading tendencies) rather than aim to rid them from medical discourse.

In this paper, we are particularly interested in the potentially misleading consequences of the metaphor of 'brain reading' or 'reading X in the brain', which is closely related to the metaphor of seeing. As stated above, Godart explicitly suggests that a perfect seeing of the brain with "good" (presumably, well-trained) eyes or vision-enhancing technologies (a "perfect microscope capable of seeing"), is part of what is necessary to read the brain (Godart 1755: 209–210). However, as Godart recognized, seeing is distinguishable from reading even if seeing is necessary for the process of reading the brain. This distinction, to which we now turn, needs further exploration to better understand the lineage and import of the 'readability-of-the-brain' metaphor.

Analytically speaking, a doctor reads a patient's charts and lab reports, but it would be wrong, except in a metaphorical sense, to speak of a doctor as reading the patient's body. However, in the case of brain imaging, it seems fitting to say that the neurologist can read the thoughts or mental states in the brain of a patient with the aid of, for example, an fMRI machine. Accordingly, it will be useful to establish some basic distinctions between seeing and reading in the medical context, both to develop a clearer idea of why the metaphor of reading has been selected in recent scholarship and because of the degree of confusion in the current use of these metaphors. That is to say, several references to reading the brain borrow some of their rhetorical force from the metaphor of seeing. Moreover, as Michel Foucault shows, the metaphor of seeing often overlaps with that of reading, where the key point of differentiation is the degree to which interpretation or mediation is required. Yet, since every reading is also a seeing in a meaningful way and vice versa, there is a potential distortive element to both metaphors.

In his 1963 work *The Birth of the Clinic*, Michel Foucault analyses the role that the metaphors of seeing and reading have played in medicine. He describes his approach as archaeological because he sifts through layers of historical documents and artefacts in order to retrace the development of medical concepts and practices, paying special attention to the relationship between medical discourse and other social phenomena, discourses, and events. Foucault attributes the development of a privileged role for seeing (which he calls the 'medical gaze') to innovations of a scientific and social nature that occurred during and after the French Revolution. In this time of great turmoil, when the university teaching of medicine was abandoned in favour of hospital-based clinical instruction, the body was reconceptualised as a three-dimensional space of tissues whose 'darkness' could be 'illuminated' by those who had the proper expertise and training (Foucault 1994: 165–166). In addition to hospital reforms and the intensification of autopsy studies, the cultivation of such an eye depended on a series of new developments, foremost among them being the discovery of different tissue morphologies by Xavier Bichat in 1802 (Bichat 1813), the rediscovery of the pathological anatomy of Giovanni Battista Morgagni (1761), and the refinement of clinical examination, as illustrated by René-Théophile-Hyacinthe Laennec's introduction of the stethoscope in 1819 (Laennec 1979).

Prior to this change in focus, eighteenth-century medicine in Europe was guided by the aim of reading the body of the patient in order to decipher the traces of disease entities that seemed to exist independently of the patient and could be ordered into types or natural kinds that were fundamentally analogous to plant and animal species, as outlined in more detail below. However, when this nosological approach to the interpretation of symptoms gave way to the search for visible lesions, the metaphor of reading soon gave way to that of seeing, as represented by the perceptive 'gaze' of the physician. Unlike reading, then, which takes time and requires an interpretive framework (i.e., a language), the act of seeing is a kind of intuitive grasp of what is immediately present. As Foucault explains:

> The glance is of the non-verbal order of *contact*, a purely ideal contact perhaps, but in fact a more *striking* contact, since it traverses more easily, and goes further beneath things. The clinical eye discovers a kinship with a new sense that prescribes its norm and epistemological structure; this is no longer the ear straining to catch a language, but the index finger palpating the depths. Hence the metaphor of 'touch' (*le tact*) by which doctors will ceaselessly define their glance. (Foucault 1994: 122)

The essential element of such a glance is that it is immediate, like touching (ignoring for the moment the fact that touching involves the rapid relay of neural signals from the finger to the brain and back). However, the tendency of this metaphor to distort lies in the fact that the eye of the physician must first be trained through extensive experience and training. The art of seeing must be cultivated, making seeing a kind of 'instantaneous reading' based on past experience and training (i. e., reading the 'signs' in the encounter). Nevertheless, the metaphor does accurately capture the idea that the exercise of judgment in context is required. That is to say, one cannot substitute an algorithmic calculation process (e. g., a computer program) for the physician who relies on instinct as well as experience when consulting a patient.

Although more closely related than it may initially seem, the metaphors of seeing and reading may be distinguished based on the degree of mediation that each requires. Reading requires the most mediation as it presupposes a syntax, grammar, code or algorithm against which what is seen must be interpreted. As a result of this necessary processing, there is a serious risk that unintended significations may be imported either through error (i. e., misreading or misapplication of the code) or as the result of the ambiguity inherent in language. For example, unless one knows English, one may see words but one cannot be said to read them. Yet, even if one speaks English fluently, the associations that attach to the words that are read will vary with each individual. In its idealized, rationalistic form, however, the metaphor of 'reading nature' assumes that the secrets of nature are written out like a language that can be understood by anyone who reads it. Moreover, this natural grammar in turn corresponds to the grammar of our own conceptual language(s), which enables us to conduct an exhaustive reading of the natural world and to impose order and predictability onto it (or rather, to see the order that is already there) (Foucault 1994: 165).

Foucault traces the origins of the reading metaphor in eighteenth-century medicine to a particular interpretation of Étienne Bonnot de Condillac's philosophy of language and to a nosological framework for explaining the nature of disease. Fundamentally, nosology at this time presupposed that diseases are classifiable according to their essential natures by analogy with the classification of animals and plants according to their species-typical characteristics. In a complex historical and philosophical analysis that requires more elucidation than the scope of this paper allows, Foucault outlines the way that symptoms are interpreted as signs whose meaning is determined in relation to a differential context or system of possible significations. That is to say, the manner in which patient symptoms refer to disease entities is analogous to the way that the letters of the alphabet convey meaning when ordered into words and sentences according to a determinate set of syntactical and grammatical rules (Foucault 1994: 117–20). The main criteria for the study of disease were the difference between symptoms as well as their timing: for example, whether the symptoms are successive or simultaneous (Foucault 1994: 93). A great nosology or 'encyclopaedia' of disease types could therefore be created based on the unique set of symptoms/signs that were presented by the disease through the patient. The interpretation of diseases thus required that the patient be abstracted from his or her case history in order to determine the essential, universal properties of the disease. Moreover, this abstraction guided the creation of the early teaching clinics (such as in Edinburgh) that sought to expose medical students to a '*structured nosological field*' that resembled a 'garden' of diseases (Foucault 1994: 59). While Foucault sees the construction of nosologies as a misreading of Condillac's philosophy, it nevertheless articulates the underlying aspiration of this dominant eighteenth-century view: namely,

> At last, there emerges on the horizon of clinical experience the possibility of an exhaustive, clear, and complete reading: for a doctor whose skills would be carried "to the highest degree of perfection, all symptoms would become signs", all pathological manifestations would speak a clear, ordered language. (Foucault 1994: 94–5)

However, even though it reflected a commitment to an abstract model of disease, Foucault shows that the seeds for a new conception of pathology and a new organization of the clinic were already taking root in this project of nosography. That is to say, the difficulties encountered during the effort to write nosologies would ultimately redirect the attention of the physician to the patient and to the importance of seeing the effects of disease on the patient's physiology.

The 'new' clinics that were created in the wake of the French Revolution did not have a teaching function in the strict sense; they were sites of research and innovation. The vast scale of new hospitals such as the École de Santé in Paris meant that physicians were exposed to a wide range of diseases and to variations of each disease that did not lend themselves to neat categorization according to rigorous nosological categories. Instead, it became essential to pay closer attention to the unique features of individual cases and to employ probabilistic reasoning to manage the uncertainty that characterised the variations in the presentation and progress of symptoms in different patients (Foucault 1994: 97–8). The irony is that Bichat, the man who articulated this new model of pathology best by means of the differentiation of tissues, was actually guided by Pinel's nosological perspective (Foucault 1994: 102). Nevertheless, Bichat's metaphor of seeing into the depths of tissues provided a new 'window' into physiology and pathology that ultimately replaced the reading metaphor (Foucault 1994: 102). Although Foucault's analysis appears to rigorously distinguish seeing and reading, he is also careful to show how these metaphors may also shift their meaning depending on the context in which they are used. There is a degree of flexibility in metaphors that may work to our advantage but may also lead to conceptual slippage or loss of meaning. For example, seeing cannot always be distinguished so easily from reading given that direct perception still presupposes a schema or framework within which what is seen needs to be interpreted. To revisit the former example, if one speaks English as a native speaker, one often just sees the meaning of words (e. g., as one approaches a STOP sign) and it is possible to forget that one is actually reading very quickly. Moreover, seeing and reading both involve the use of other senses that seem to deviate from the metaphor: for example, reading in Braille substitutes touch for sight and one can of course listen to a public reading or lecture. However, seeing 'happens' in an instant when one opens one's eyes, or at least it seems to if one ignores the series of interpretive acts that occur (not least of which is the inversion of the image transmitted from the eye to the brain). By contrast, reading takes longer and requires a code or language that is more explicitly dependent on interpretation than is the seeing of objects or colours, for example. Still, the dream of 'reading nature' has not died out and its effects are still uncertain. That is to say, the pressure to restate novel medical possibilities in terms that are already at hand threatens to distort their meaning and limit the possibility of what may yet be achieved, notwithstanding the benefits it may also bring.

3. POSSIBLE MISLEADING EFFECTS
OF THE 'BRAIN-READING' METAPHOR

Thus far we have been concerned to survey the ambiguities of the readability metaphor, drawing from the history of science and medicine, paying special attention to the sixteenth through nineteenth centuries. Next we investigated more closely how metaphors may be confusing when used in medicine in general. Now we will look at how the readability metaphor is employed more specifically in the context of contemporary neuroimaging research and its relevant applications, bearing in mind how the historical freight of this terminology both augments and constrains our understanding of the relevant findings.

According to the *Merriam Webster Dictionary* – much like the definition from the *Oxford English Dictionary* given above – a metaphor is "a figure of speech in which a word or phrase literally denoting one kind of object or idea is used in place of another to suggest a likeness or analogy between them (as in *drowning in money*)" (Merriam-Webster 2010). Perelman and Olbrechts-Tyteca have noted that in the context of argumentation, metaphors act as condensed analogies. Aristotle shows this explicitly in the *Poetics* (XXI: 1457b) with the following example: "As old age is to life, so is evening to day. One will accordingly describe evening as the 'old age of the day' and old age as the 'evening of life'" (quoted in Perelman & Olbrechts-Tyteca 1969: 399, nt. 179). Perelman and Olbrechts-Tyteca have analyzed the structural relations of Aristotle's example, noting that it demonstrates a logic whereby "'A is to B as C is to D' yields the expression 'C of B' to designate A." (Perelman & Olbrechts-Tyteca 1969: 399). So also, we can say that: "(A) Neuroimaging is to (B) the brain, as (C) reading is to (D) symbolic expression (e.g. written language)". Accordingly, this yields the expression 'reading of the brain' ('C of B') to designate (A) neuroimaging. It is important to remember, however, that metaphors are a kind of trope, and as Quintilian explains in *The Institutio Oratoria* (VIII, VI, 1) a trope involves "'the artistic alteration of a word or phrase from its proper meaning to another'" (quoted in Perelman & Olbrechts-Tyteca 1969: 398–399, nt. 174). Since metaphors are commonly used as rhetorical figures of speech (that achieve their effects via analogy), we need to further probe how the analogies between reading and modern neuroimaging built into the 'brain-reading' metaphor rightfully explain or potentially obfuscate the meaning of reported findings achieved through neuroimaging. With this in mind, we turn now to a discussion of contemporary neuroimaging and the discourses surrounding it.

Modern neuroimaging technologies – for example, computed axial tomography (CT), diffuse optical imaging (DOI), event-related optical signal (EROS), magnetic resonance imaging (MRI), functional magnetic resonance imaging (fMRI), electroencephalography (EEG), magnetoencephalography (MEG), positron emission tomography (PET), and single photon emission computed tomography (SPECT) – hold out an unprecedented promise of medical innovation (Logothetis & Wandell 2004). Even if these imaging technologies are not restricted to neurological applications, some have been used to provide structural imaging of the brain, for the purposes of diagnosing larger-scale intracranial diseases, tumours, injuries, and stroke. Others have been used to provide functional imaging of the brain, used for various purposes including: i) the diagnosis of smaller tumours, lesions, and diseases (e. g. metabolic diseases) on a finer scale; as well as, ii) brain mapping for research into neurological and cognitive psychology that correlates brain areas with specific functions (Haberfeld et al. 2010). With the latter expansive applications of the technology we are developing new ways of investigating the brain that extend far beyond clinical purposes to correlate mental or psychological states to physical (i. e. brain) states or structures (cf. Zanzotto & Croce 2010).

As it stands, many neuroscientists and certain neurophilosophers are now talking as if the newly available technological powers for observing the brain will surely lead us to the mind – that the mind can be read from the brain (see table 1, part 2). As Kamitani and Tong write: "The potential for human neuroimaging to read out the detailed contents of a person's mental state has yet to be fully explored" (Kamitani & Tong 2005). Following this hope, Haynes and colleagues purport to use brain scans to "decod[e] mental states from brain activity in humans" (Haynes & Rees 2006). Friston further claims that, "all demonstrations of functionally specialized responses – demonstrating a significant mapping between mental states and brain signals – represent an implicit mind reading" (Friston 2009; cf. De Charms 2008).

The arc of Godart's eighteenth-century theory – that claims that the brain holds inscribed within itself the whole of an individual's personal history – clearly traces through to present-day conceptions that apply correlation analyses to investigate the readability potential of the brain. We see evidence of this in talk of "decoding" the brain for mental contents (Kamitani & Tong 2005), and finding in it "neural signatures" or "neural codes" (see table 1, part 3). Modern neuroimaging technologies also carry forward the impetus of Godart to open the brain for viewing, and like a text, read from it the language contained therein. What is new with these technologies, as compared with the instruments for investigation in previous epochs is the capacity to, as one textbook puts it, "see inside and 'read' a *living* human brain" (emphasis added), and to do so with increasing sophistication (Haberfeld et al. 2010). But as Watson points out, "Bridging the gap between understanding the brain and understanding the mind and behaviour continues to elude us" (Watson 1996: 544). Even so, the belief in the readability of the brain by way of modern neuroimaging techniques seems to trace forward Godart's belief that we are closing this gap, first "with very good eyes", then with the promise of "the perfect microscope", and now with instruments of much greater accuracy as available through modern neuroimaging (see table 1, part 2).

However, Godart's "very good eyes" or, as the case may be, neuroimaging technology that can "perfect" our powers of vision, count as examples of sight, and sight counts as a pre-requisite for most kinds of reading (Braille, being an exception to this norm). But, to repeat, powers of vision, no matter how accurate, are insufficient by themselves to make reading possible: as Godart also noted, it is not enough to be able to see the imprinting of the "letters" of thought in the brain (cf. Willingham & Dunn 2003); also needed is "an ability to comprehend their signification" (Godart 1755: 208–210). Is neuroimaging, then, better described as a practice in 'seeing', as opposed to 'reading', the brain? Answering this question, as we shall see, can indirectly also answer our query as to the limitations of the 'brain-reading' metaphor.

A proper answer to the question at hand hinges on what kind of reading is implied. On the one hand, the practice of reading as applied to texts like laws, works of art (e. g. plays, novels) or newspapers all involve a great deal of interpretation on the part of the reader to produce understanding. On the other hand, the term 'reading' can also be used to describe "data indicated by an instrument" (Merriam-Webster 2010) as we would speak of, for example, 'a meter reading', or 'a temperature reading'. To read the latter sort of 'read-outs' obviously involves comparatively little (thought arguably still *some*) interpretation. Reading of this kind would almost be akin to near 'instantaneous reading' of a STOP sign – that is to say, reading practices that are so routine that they have veritably become non-conscious or unconscious. As stated above, Foucault has shown that the metaphor of 'seeing' often overlaps with that of 'reading', where the key point of differentiation is the degree to which interpretation or mediation is required. So where reading involves very little interpretation and therefore involves minimal cognitive processing, it becomes like seeing. Insofar as the metaphor 'reading the brain' is used to designate modern neuroimaging practices, where the 'reading' involved is understood as requiring a great deal of interpretation, the use of the trope seems valid. In the act of reading a sentence (as with reading a language), one observes letters but seeing them *as* letters that form words whose ordering delineate sentences that signify propositions requires *seeing* beyond and past the surface appearance of scratches on the page. So also 'reading the brain' with neuroimaging is much more than a matter of straightforward observation.

Michael Coles, in an article entitled 'Modern Mind-Brain Reading' surmises that "[p]sychophysiological measures, particularly those of the event-related brain potential … can serve as 'windows' on the mind and as 'windows' on the brain" (see Coles 1989). Yet, this idea does not reflect the real possibilities offered by new neurotechnologies. Moreover, the 'window' metaphor adds to the confusion because it implies that one can just see the brain even though such 'seeing' is in fact a reading. That is to say, a technological device is required to 'open' that window using sophisticated computer programming to read the data. After all, the results of fMRI, for example, rely on computer processing based on algorithms derived from statistical comparisons that are used to generate images that approximate representations of brain functioning. On a popular and cultural understanding, neuroimaging technologies can be applied from the outside of a subject to represent (or mirror) the interior of the subject (Kevles 1997; cf. De Charms 2008). This commitment assumes that images stand in for something more fundamental of which they are technological copies (Van Dijck 2005). However, most modern imaging technologies do not operate as x-rays do (Doby & Alker 1997). The images are not to be confused with accurate representations, but rather approximate configurations, producing meaningful correlates rather than a mirror of the reality of what is imaged. As such, they are types of description that act, not as observations, but as ciphers requiring interpretation by physicians and neuroimagists.

In this regard, the 'brain-reading' metaphor effectively captures the highly-mediated nature of neuroimaging in relation to the relevant living brain that is being imaged. Insofar as the metaphor 'reading the brain' is used to designate modern neuroimaging practices, where the sense of 'reading' that is implied is much like that when reading a text of some sort, the metaphor seems to be valid. However, insofar as the 'brain-reading' metaphor is taken to imply the kind of reading involved when removing information from an automatic device (e. g. water meter read-out, or computer read-out), it denies the interpretive aspects of the process and in this regard the trope is potentially very misleading. Greater powers of 'seeing' may seem available to us through modern neuroimaging, but the greater accuracy of representations have not obviated the interpretive element for determining findings of tumours, lesions, and diseases in the brain, let alone findings for such things as "intentions", "thoughts", "the will" (Haggard 2008), or "'the mind".

As outlined above with regard to the power of metaphors, it is essential to reflect on the history or genealogy of metaphors in order to be able to use them wisely. The often implicit (or hidden) meaning(s) of metaphors may serve to distort reality or limit our capacity to chart new directions and to make sense of the research findings. Even the metaphor of reading, as distinct from seeing, admits of two different senses that are often run together in the neuroscientific literature and in popular literature. That is to say, the expression 'brain reading' or 'reading X in the brain' crystallizes relatively dissimilar expectations. The more restrictive scope of what in the brain presents itself for reading, to which actual neuroscientific findings correspond, should be rigorously distinguished from the more expansive scope of what the brain presents for reading, to which representations and fantasies (supposedly) correspond. In other words, the process of collecting brain data is often confused with reading as a cognitive process of decoding symbols (an interpretive process) that is effectively analogous to making sense of expressions of a language.

The 'brain-reading' metaphor in itself is not responsible for this confusion. Indeed it might be even worse if we were to routinely speak and write of 'seeing X in the brain' as opposed to 'reading X in the brain'. At the very least, the trope of reading conveys the important need for interpretation to make sense of the findings of (data produced by) neuroimaging technologies. But treating the brain as if it were a subject to be read – a veritable linguistic entity – as opposed to an object to be observed, is potentially misleading. Doing so, and with the routine use and entrenchment of the metaphor, we sometimes forget that it is only a metaphor and come to believe that our observations of the brain through neuroimaging provide anything more than data; instead these 'readings of the brain' are made to assume a certain symbolic status, entrenching a belief in metaphysical notions like the mind (see table 1, part 2), just as scratches on a page signify words that stand in for concepts or ideas.

4. CONCLUSIONS

There is currently a discrepancy within the domain of neuroimaging technologies between what is induced by hyperbole (including talk of being able 'to *read* X in the brain') and what is concretely possible through science and medicine. The explicit reading of an individual's accumulated experience (i. e. mental states, personality, intentions, memories, etc), for instance, is still very far from being possible today. Quite the contrary, neuroscientists and physicians are among the first to admit the extent of what remains unexplained in brain functioning. For this reason, even the diagnostic use of brain scans remains problematic. Although researchers are able to, for example, see the brain's bioelectrical activity in relation to specific goal-related tasks carried out in laboratories and have software that recognizes certain predefined paths of cerebral activity, this highly mediated and technological act of 'reading' stands in stark contrast to some of the hyped promises for this technology: e. g., to detect lying (Thompson 2005; cf. De Charms 2008: 724; Fenton et al. 2009; Ireland 2007; Kerr et al. 2008; Langleben et al. 2002; Langleben 2008; Spence et al. 2004), criminal intent (Barrie 2008; West 2007; cf. Khoshbin & Khoshbin 2007; Krahn et al. 2009; Marks 2007; Morse 2006) or the lack thereof (Hartocollis 2007; cf. Appelbaum 2009).

New technology brings new ways of thinking about neuroscience and medicine. These new ways of thinking may be shaped by the way that we talk about new developments. Where we are forced to draw on older metaphors that are inappropriate or inaccurate, a distortion may result. This is especially true when the metaphor is used uncritically or without due appreciation of its scope and impact. Neuroscientists and physicians must resort to the use of terms already laden with meaning, and often burdened by tradition, at the risk of importing through these words connotations that do not tally with the sought-after objectivity of empirical science. The use of the readability metaphor carries with it both positive and negative consequences. We do not condemn the 'brain-reading' metaphor *per* se as used to discuss the practice of neuroimaging. To be fair, the 'brain-reading' metaphor as an explanation of neuroimaging is not without merit since it makes accessible for a multiplicity of stakeholders what we otherwise find very difficult to describe in nontechnical language, and it speaks to the explicit interpretive elements germane to the technology. The distortion occurs when the metaphor is understood not as a figurative form of speech – "an artistic alteration of a word or phrase from its proper meaning", to quote Quintilian (1920:VIII, vi, 1) – but is instead taken literally, not as a metaphor. In effect this sets up the brain as a text or linguistic subject which then fuels expectations to find by way of neuroimaging technologies evidence of metaphysical entities that are (not surprisingly) not empirically observable. Though historical precedents explain some of the sources and traditions that underwrite the sensibility of 'brain-reading' metaphor as it has its life in discussions of modern neuroimaging technologies, we do well to critically check certain distortions (even false expectations) carried forward from the past that are also bundled with the use of this way of speaking (and writing) about the brain.

ACKNOWLEDGEMENT

Thanks to Alexandre Wenger for enlightening discussions which were invaluable to us in drafting the argument of this paper. Thanks to Françoise Baylis and the Novel Tech Ethics research team for feedback on earlier drafts. Research for this project has been funded by Canadian Institutes of Health Research, MOP 77670, Therapeutic Hopes and ethical concerns: Clinical research in the neurosciences and by Canadian Institutes of Health Research, NNF 80045, States of Mind: Emerging Issues in Neuroethics.

REFERENCES

Ackerknecht, E. H. (1968) 'A Short History of Medicine' (New York, NY: Ronald Press Co.).

Amodio, D. M. & C. D. Frith (2006) 'Meeting of Minds: The Medial Frontal Cortex and Social Cognition', Nature Reviews Neuroscience 7(4): 268–277.

Anonymous (2006) 'What's on Your Mind?', Nature Neuroscience 9(8): 981.

Anonymous (2009) 'Abstractions', Nature 458(7238): 548.

Appelbaum, P. S. (2009) 'Law & Psychiatry: Through a Glass Darkly: Functional Neuroimaging Evidence Enters the Courtroom', Psychiatric Services 60(1): 21–23.

Barrie, A. (2008) 'Homeland Security Detects Terrorist Threats by Reading Your Mind'. Source: FoxNews.com. http://www.foxnews.com/printer_friendly_story/0,3566,426485,00.html. Accessed 15 November 2010.

Bichat, X. (1813) 'A Treatise on The Membranes in General, and of Different Membranes in Particular' (A new edition, enlarged by an historical notice of the life and writings of the author, by M. Husson, Paris, 1802. Translated by J. G. Coffin. Boston, MA: Cummings and Hilliard).

Blumenberg, H. (1981) 'Die Lesbarkeit der Welt' (Frankfurt am Main: Suhrkamp).

Childress, J. F. (1997) 'Practical Reasoning in Bioethics' (Bloomington, IL: Indiana University Press).

Coles, M. G. H. (1989) 'Modern Mind-Brain Reading – Psychophysiology, Physiology, and Cognition', Psychophysiology 26(3): 251–269.

Conti, F. & G. Corbellini (2008) 'Italian Neuroscientists are Ready to start the Debate', Nature 451(7179): 627.

Daston, L. & P. Galison (2007) 'Objectivity' (Cambridge, MA: MIT Press).

De Charms, R. C. (2008) 'Applications of Real-Time fMRI', Nature Reviews Neuroscience 9(9): 720–729.

Doby, T. & G. J. Alker (1997) 'Origins and Development of Medical Imaging' (Carbondale, IL: Southern Illinois University Press).

Eamon, W. (1994) 'Science and the Secrets of Nature: Books of Secrets in Medieval and Early Modern Culture' (Princeton, NJ: Princeton University Press).

Fenton, A., L. Meynell & F. Baylis (2009) *'Ethical Challenges and Interpretive Difficulties with Non-Clinical Applications of Pediatric fMRI'*, The American Journal of Bioethics 9(1): 3–13.

Foucault, M. (1994) *'The Birth of the Clinic: An Archaeology of Medical Perception'* (Translated by A. M. Sheridan. New York, NY: Vintage Books).

Friston, K. J. (2009) *'Modalities, Modes, and Models in Functional Neuroimaging'*, Science 326(5951): 399 403.

Galilei, G. (1957) *'Discoveries and Opinions of Galileo'* (Translated by S. Drake. New York, NY: Anchor Books).

Godart, G-L. (1755) *'La Physique de l'Âme humaine. Par Mr. Godart, Docteur en Médecine'* (Berlin: Aux dépens de la Compagnie).

Golinski, J. (2005) *'Making Natural Knowledge: Constructivism and the History of Science'* (Chicago, IL: University of Chicago Press).

Goodman, K. (2000) *'The Reading Process'*, in P. L. Carrell, J. Devine & D. E. Eskey (eds), *Interactive Approaches to Second Language Reading* (London & New York, NY: Cambridge University Press: 11–21).

Haberfeld, E., J. Seidenfeld, D. J. Feivelson & R. L. Fischbach (2010) *'Neuroimaging: Visualizing Brain Structure and Function'*. Source: *Center for Bioethics at the College of Physicians and Surgeons* of Columbia University. http://ccnmtl.columbia.edu/projects/neuroethics/module1/foundationtext/index.html. Accessed 15 November 2010.

Hacking, I. (2007) *'Representing and Intervening: Introductory Topics in the Philosophy of Natural Science'* (Cambridge, MA: Cambridge University Press).

Haggard, P. (2008) *'Human Volition: Towards a Neuroscience of Will'*, Nature Reviews Neuroscience 9(12): 934–946.

Hartocollis, A. (2007) *'In Support of Sex Attacker's Insanity Plea, a Look at His Brain'*. Source: *The New York Times* (online). http://query.nytimes.com/gst/fullpage.html?res=940DE6D61431F93 2A25756C0A9619C8B3. Accessed 15 November 2010.

Haynes, J. D. & G. Rees. (2006) *'Decoding Mental States from Brain Activity in Humans'*, Nature Reviews Neuroscience 7(7): 523–534.

Hutson, S. (2005) *'Our Bodies as We Have Never Seen Them Before'*, New Scientist 188(2530): 26–29.

Ireland, C. (2007) *'Symposium: "Will Brain Imaging Be Lie Detector Test of the Future?"'* Source: Harvard Gazette. http://news.harvard.edu/gazette/story/2007/02/symposium-will brain-imaging-be-lie-detector-test-of-the-future/. Accessed 15 November 2010.

Kamitani, Y. & F. Tong (2005) *'Decoding the Visual and Subjective Contents of the Human Brain'*, Nature Neuroscience 8(5): 679–685.

Kay, K. N., T. Naselaris, R. J. Prenger & J. L. Gallant (2008) *'Identifying Natural Images From Human Brain Activity'*, Nature 452(7185): 352–3U7.

Kerr, I., M. Binnie & C. Aoki (2008) *'Tessling On My Brain: The Future of Lie Detection and Brain Privacy in the Criminal Justice System'*, Canadian Journal of Criminology and Criminal Justice 50(3): 367–387.

Kevles, B. H. (1997) *'Naked to the Bone: Medical Imaging in the Twentieth Century'* (New Brunswick, NJ: Rutgers University Press).

Krahn, T., A. Fenton & L. Meynell (2009) *'Novel Neurotechnologies in Film – A Reading of Steven Spielberg's Minority Report'*, Neuroethics 3(1): 73–88.

Laennec, R. T. H. (1979) *'A Treatise on the Diseases of the Chest in Which They are Described According to Their anatomical Characters, and Their Diagnosis Established on a New Principle by Means of Acoustick Instruments'* (Translated by J. Forbes. Birmingham, AL: Classics of Medicine Library).

Lakoff, G. & M. Johnson (1980) *Metaphors We Live By* (Chicago, IL: University of Chicago Press).

Langleben, D. D. (2008) *'Detection of Deception with fMRI: Are We There Yet?'* Legal and Criminological Psychology 13: 1–9.

Langleben, D. D., L. Schroeder, J. A. Maldjian, R. C. Gur, S. McDonald, J. D. Ragland et al. (2002) *'Brain Activity During Simulated Deception: An Event-Related Functional Magnetic Resonance Study'*, Neuroimage 15(3): 727–732.

Le Camus, A., L.É. Ganeau & H. S.-P. Gissey. (1760) *'Mémoires sur Divers Sujets de Médecine. Et sur le Cerveau, Principe de la Génération'* (Paris: chez Ganeau, libraire).

Logothetis, N. K. & B. A. Wandell (2004) *'Interpreting the BOLD Signal'*, Annual Review of Physiology 66: 735–769.

Martensen, R. L. (2004) *'The Brain Takes Shape: An Early History'* (New York, NY: Oxford University Press).

Marks, J. H. (2007) *'Interrogational Neuroimaging in Counterterrorism: A "no-brainer" or a Human Rights Hazard?'* American Journal of Law & Medicine 33(2/3): 483–500.

Martinez-Conde, S. & S. L. Macknik (2007) *'Windows On the Mind'*, Scientific American 297(2): 56–63.

Merriam-Webster (2010) *'Merriam-Webster online dictionary'*. Source: 2010 Merriam Webster, Incorporated. http://www.merriam-webster.com/. Accessed 15 November 2010.

Morgagni, G. (1761) *'De Sedibus, et Causis Morborum per Anatomen Indagatis Libri Quinque. Dissectiones, et Animadversiones, Nunc Primum Editas, Complectuntur Propemodum Innumeras, Medicis, Chirurgis, Anatomicis Profuturas. Multiplex Praefixus est Index Rerum, & Nominum Accoratissimus'* (Venetiis: Extypographia Remondiniana).

Morse, S. J. (2006) *'Brain Overclaim Syndrome and Criminal Responsbility: A Diagnostic Note'*, Ohio State Journal of Criminal Law 3: 397–412.

OED (2010) *'Oxford English Dictionary (online)'*. Source: Oxford University Press 2010. http://www.oed.com/. Accessed 15 November 2010.

Op de Beeck, H. P., J. Haushofer & N. G. Kanwisher (2008) *'Interpreting fMRI Data: Maps, Modules and Dimensions'*, Nature Reviews Neuroscience 9(2): 123–135.

Owen, A. M. & M. R. Coleman (2008) *'Functional Neuroimaging of the Vegetative State'*, Nature Reviews Neuroscience 9(3): 235–243.

Pearson, H. (2006) *'Lure of Lie Detectors Spooks Ethicists'*, Nature 441(7096): 918–919.

Peirce, C. S. (1998) *'What is a sign?'* in N. Houser, A. De Teienne, J. R. Eller, C. L. Clark, A. C. Lewis & D. Bront Davis (eds), The Essential Peirce: Selected Philosophical Writings – Volume 2 (Peirce Edition Project. Bloomington and Indianapolis, IN: Indiana University Press: 4–10).

Perelman, C. & L. Olbrechts-Tyteca. 1969. *'The New Rhetoric: A Treatise on Argumentation'* (Notre Dame, IN: University of Notre Dame Press).

Quintilian (1920) *'The Institutio Oratoria of Quintilian'* (Translated and edited by H. E. Butler. London: W. Heinemann).

Rabinowitz, P. J. (1998) *'Before Reading: Narrative Conventions and the Politics of Interpretation'* (Columbus OH: Ohio State University Press).

Sawday, J. (1995) *'The Body Emblazoned: Dissection and the Human Body in Renaissance Culture'* (London: Routledge).

Schrock, K. (2007) *'Freeing a Locked-In Mind'*, Scientific American Mind 18: 40–45.

Sismondo, S. (2010) *'An Introduction to Science and Technology Studies'* (2nd ed. Chichester, West Sussex, UK: Wiley-Blackwell).

Smith, C. U. M. (2010) *'Understanding the Nervous System in the 18th Century'*, in J. A. Michael (ed), Handbook of Clinical Neurology: History of Neurology – Volume 95 (Edinburgh: Elsevier: 107–114).

Smith, K. (2008) *'Mind-Reading with a Brain Scan'*. Source: NatureNews. http://www.nature.com/news/2008/080305/full/news.2008.650.html. Accessed 15 November 2010.

Spence, S. A., M. D. Hunter, T. F. Farrow, R. D. Green, D. H. Leung, C. J. Hughes et al. (2004) *'A Cognitive Neurobiological Account of Deception: Evidence from Functional Neuroimaging'*, Philosophical Transactions of the Royal Society B: Biological Science 359(1451): 1755–1762.

Stefansson, H. (2007) *'The Biology of Behaviour: Scientific and Ethical Implications – Introduction'*, EMBO Reports 8: S1–S2.

Thompson, S. K. (2005) *'The Legality of the Use of Psychiatric Neuroimaging in Intelligence Inter-rogation'*, *Cornell Law Review* 90(6): 1601–1637.

Van Dijck, J. (2005) *The Transparent Body: A cultural Analysis of Medical Imaging* (Seattle, WA: University of Washington Press).

Vesalius, A. (1998) *On the Fabric of the Human Body. Book I, The Bones and Cartilages* (Translated by W. F. Richardson in collaboration with J. B. Carman. San Francisco, CA: Norman Publishing).

Von Staden, H. (1995) *'Anatomy as Rhetoric: Galen on Dissection and Persuasion'*, *Journal of the History of Medicine and Allied Sciences* 50(1): 47–66.

Waldby, C. (2000) *'Virtual Anatomy: From the Body in the Text to the Body on the Screen'*, *Journal of Medical Humanities* 21(2): 85–107.

Watson, D. B. (1996) *'Opening the Doors – Looking Back to Move Forward'*, *Canadian Journal of Psychiatry Revue Canadienne de Psychiatrie* 41(9): 543–548.

Wegner, A. & F. Gilbert (2007) *'Le Cerveau à Livre Ouvert'*, *Revue Médicale Suisse* 3: 2564–2566.

West, P. (2007) 'The nightmare of "pre-crime"'. Source: SPECTATOR.CO.UK. http://www.spectator.co.uk/essays/all/313761/the-nightmare-of-precrime-is-already-with-us.thtml. Accessed 15November 2010.

Willingham, D. T. & E. W. Dunn (2003) *'What Neuroimaging and Brain Localization Can Do, Cannot Do, and Should Not Do for Social Psychology'*, *Journal of Personality and Social Psychology* 85(4): 662–671.

Wilson, C. (1995) *'The Invisible World: Early Modern Philosophy and the Invention of the Microscope.'* (Princeton, N. J: Princeton University Press).

Zanzotto, F. M. & D. Croce (2010) *'Comparing EEG/ERP-Like and fMRI-Like Techniques for Reading Machine Thoughts'*, in Y. Yao, R. Sun, T. Poggio, J. Liu, N. Zhong & J. Huang (eds), *Brain Informatics: International Conference, BI 2010,* Toronto, ON, Canada, August 28–30, 2010: *Conference Proceedings* (Berlin: Springer: 133–144).

Zwart, H. (1998) *'Medicine, Symbolization and the "Real" Body – Lacan's Understanding of Medical Science'*, *Medicine Health Care and Philosophy* 1(2): 107–117.

NEUROIMAGI(NI)NG IN PAST AND PRESENT – REPRESENTATION, EPISTEMOLOGY AND CIRCULATORY REFERENCES

Heiner Fangerau, Robert Lindenberg

ABSTRACT

Visualization of the human brain and representations of its functional state play a prominent role in contemporary neuroscience research. The present paper aims to elucidate the process of imaging and imagining the brain from three perspectives: (a) visualization and the cultural techniques of producing images; (b) the historical context of neuroimages; and (c) the insight afforded into current research and analysis methods. The concept of circulatory references, proposed by Bruno Latour, serves as a heuristic guideline to illustrate the interconnectedness of representation and epistemological processes. Special emphasis is placed on the epistemological status of functional "digital images" compared to traditional imaging techniques.

IMAGINING THE BRAIN

It has become a truism that we can only see what we know (Fleck, 1983 [1947]). Every student of anatomy – microscopic or macroscopic – must learn a *pictorial vocabulary* to gain the ability to differentiate structures. The view under a microscope may appear as a meaningless, unstructured coloured picture to the untrained eye. Similarly, cerebral components of the brain may appear indistinguishable. Early descriptions compared the appearance of the brain to that of the lower intestines and later, gyri were even described as having the appearance of a plate of macaroni (Clarke and Dewhurst, 1996, p. 65).

For many years descriptions of the brain surface remained vague. Until the 16th century illustrations of the brain emphasized the ventricles, which at the time were considered to host the soul. Hence, the ventricles were the only intracranial structures depicted in detail. Illustrators abstracted from first aspects, natural appearance or "reality" by placing their drawings into a common theory concerning the assumed role and function of the brain. The rediscovery of the dissection method was crucial for this development (Gombrich, 1987, pp. 77–99; Sawday, 1995). "Dissection" was so named due to the necessity of destroying the surface of the body to gain insights into the mechanisms of interacting structures.

During the Renaissance, many doctrines concerning science and society were challenged, and anatomy was not exempt. Until the 15th century, clinging to the principles of Galenic medicine, doctors did not see the need to perform dissections.

With the re-appraisal of antiquated theories came the idea of using human dissections to gain insight into the mysteries of life. Furthermore, dissection provided access to the physicality of the brain and its structures. The inner organization of the brain became the main focus of study. The anatomist Andreas Vesalius (1514–1564), for example, systematically sliced axial cuts through the brain. Vesalius described his dissection techniques in detail so as to allow for replication, thus standardizing brain dissections. Along with a standardized approach to brain dissections was the idea of providing illustrations as visual documentation to aid in the understanding of brain anatomy. Realistic illustrations together with detailed descriptions would serve to be convincing to contemporaries and to guide fellow scientists in the replication of findings (Saunders, 1982).

Various levels of abstraction (from data to icons) were created as a means of visualizing the brain in numerous ways. Physical dissection allowed Vesalius, as one of the most prominent pioneers of new anatomy, to move from schematic diagrams, concentrating on Galenic dogmata, to virtually three-dimensional representations. While the drawings of Vesalius and others were progressive as compared to previous images, they were still bound by the technology of the time. The application of human dissection along with new techniques and instruments (e. g. the microscope) facilitated the ability to view different aspects of the cerebrum. The new images produced by these techniques provided an inside-outside, layered perspective, opening up a deeper understanding of the body. This method consisted of reducing a multi-facetted holistic view to a key-feature (Veltman and Keele, 1986, pp. 209 sqq.).

Contemporary neuroscience research has greatly benefited from the path paved by Vesalius and his followers. Current brain images fit within the framework established by the dissection method. Today, three-dimensional images of the human brain along with the ability to view the brain "at work" through *functional magnetic resonance imaging* (fMRI), *positron emission tomography* (PET), *magneto-encephalography* (MEG), and *electro-encephalography* (EEG) play a prominent role in understanding brain function. However, while the data used to generate these images are fully three-dimensional, the actual presentation of digital images follows earlier anatomical representations of dissected brains.

The connection of brain images and their theoretical background as well as the associated paradigm-shifts in the history of medicine have been examined thoroughly elsewhere (e. g. Meyer, 1971; Lantos, 1983; Clarke and Dewhurst, 1996; Breidbach, 1997; Hagner, 1997; Maudgil, 1997; Linden, 2002). Similarly, the development of symbolic representations such as the iconography of arrows to illustrate cerebral function has been analyzed (Schott, 2000). Amongst others, Illes examined the ethical challenges put forward by contemporary functional "imaging or imagining" (Illes, 2005).

Here we describe three crucial transitions in methods of generating brain images. In order to demonstrate the role of the cultural and scientific background inherent to any image of the brain, we start with a short description of the difference between "image" and "picture". We then focus on the transitions from (1) drawings to woodcuts, (2) woodcuts to radiographs, and (3) radiographs to digital imaging. A special emphasis is placed on the comparison of drawings and functional digital imaging while examining the extent to which these methods differ regarding (a) process of production, (b) epistemological impact, and (c) scientific intent.

IMAGES, PICTURES, AND "CIRCULATORY REFERENCES"

The difference between *picture* and *image* can be described by the following: a *picture* depicts visual items to display "facts", like a document. A picture reflects a fake-reality that interprets similarities. By contrast, an *image* is a symbolic representation of physical elements. Images include several symbols that serve as cultural markers, each with a designated meaning that must be learned. In opposition to common thought, these symbols are not self-explanatory. To understand images, specific codes must be deciphered or deconstructed (Rorty, 1967; Mitchell, 1986; Mitchell, 1994; Roeck, 2003). Depictions of the brain have always involved (and evolved) techniques which abstract from reality via anatomical preparation, special photo- or radiographic setting, and we thus tend to speak of *images* of the brain instead of *pictures*.

In the history of art, the role of the *spectator* is characterized by the interrelation of space *(milieu/laboratory)*, visual perception, and the construction of the image.[1] The theorist of critical iconology Erwin Panofsky contradicts an imminent perspective dissolved from a cultural context and tradition (Panofsky, 1985). Furthermore, the retrospective logical discourse that occurs when analyzing an image links individual experience with factual knowledge and opposes simple sensation-perception experience and thus cannot be determined ex-post. This theory is valid not only in art history but also holds true in the interpretation of neuroimages. Different processes of producing images of the brain involve different levels of abstraction from reality. Nevertheless, neuroscientists are able to interpret images according to their cultural setting. When viewing a brain image therefore, neuroscientists must be understood as active participants and not passive spectators. They are actively involved in image development, neurological visualization, and the interplay between theory and application. The experts/specialists "translate" images into precise descriptions of neuroscientific phenomena. Furthermore, due to their training, neuroscientists are able to recapitulate each step leading from the actual brain to the image at hand. However, in practice this ability takes the form of tacit knowledge. The technology involved is a "black box"; the developmental process of imaging is not necessarily evident. This mostly hidden process of technical visualization as well as verbal "translation" must be made conscious in order to elucidate the underpinnings of imaging and imagining the brain.

One method of making the technical, interpretative, and translational aspects of imaging the brain conscious can be derived from a model developed by the philosopher of science Bruno Latour (1999). Latour describes the creation of reality's

---

1   We are indebted to Julia Schäfer for her helpful comments and corrections with this section.

representations as "circulatory references". In several successive steps, he explains how that which is seen by the eye or found in nature is transformed into a representation. This representation is accessible in a standardized format by every scientist/ recipient accustomed to a certain mode of thinking. Thus, via a chain of representations, an initial aspect is transformed into for example, a text or an image. During this process the original subject is rendered and adapted; certain aspects are amplified or reduced. The transformation at each stage of the chain of references "may be pictured as a trade-off between what is gained [amplification] and what is lost [reduction] at each information producing step" (Latour, 1999, pp. 24–79, 71). However, an essential property of the subject must be traceable in both directions, the single transformation steps must be reversible to allow for "referencing" the subject in question to its original appearance (ibid.). Furthermore, the result of each referencing step represents the original subject's essentials, which must be highlighted by the chain's final product. Circularity is also achieved as each step captures previous or further amplifications and reductions.

In the aspect of "circulatory references" the differences in the production process of brain images gain special importance in their epistemological status and scientific/medical application. Latour illustrates the chain of references with an example from pedology. He demonstrates how a grain of soil, via several steps, is transformed into a scientific paper, including cartographic, microscopic, chemical and physical analysis reference steps and graphic display formats. Images of the brain are similarly produced along a chain of references. The chain of references is determined by the image's purpose and available techniques. The chain itself determines the interpretation of the image.

SHIFTING REFERENCES

Transition 1: From drawings to woodcuts

Early medical texts included limited imagery. Doctrines were transferred from generation to generation by words, not images. The development of the printed image in the 15th century triggered crucial changes in the imaging of the human brain (Tsafrir and Ohry, 2001). Through the invention of woodblock prints and, later, copper engravings more sophisticated and higher quality reproductions of a particular view of the brain could be disseminated among scholars. Through these reproductions, a "harmonized" image was transmitted while new ideas and new views were spread at a faster pace (Tessman and Suarez, 2002).

Leonardo da Vinci (1452–1519) was among the first to invent key techniques in the pictorial representation of the brain. These techniques shaped early widespread images of the brain during the Renaissance. Da Vinci introduced the "solid section" which displayed properties of three-dimensional images for the depiction of structures. In addition, the "exploded view", a method of displaying elements of an object slightly separated from each other was developed. His intention was to draw anatomical structures in layers in order to show their relative positions towards each other. Furthermore, da Vinci altered the perspective angles on the structures he de-picted.

In the 16th century Andreas Vesalius – the most prominent among the early anatomists using woodcuts to illustrate text – added further perspectives to brain images that remain quite stable even today. Vesalius placed axial (horizontal) cuts through the brain, a pattern replicated by twentieth century radiological approaches. The work of Vesalius was revolutionary in various aspects. Not only did he chal-lenge many of Galen's assumptions on human anatomy, he also described his method of dissection in detail so that others could replicate his results. Unlike da Vinci's depictions that were never published, Vesalius' work was printed and widely circulated.

The next level of abstraction in brain imaging was introduced by Vesalius' con-temporary Bartholomeo Eustachio (1520?–1574). Eustachio pioneered morpho-logical studies of the nervous system by abstracting his depictions from many indi-vidual anatomical observations. He did not attempt to depict precisely each indi-vidual brain studied. Instead, Eustachio combined several observations into ab-stracted "standard images" of the brain, a strategy that is applied even today. In addition, Eustachio introduced a graduated scale to accompany his diagrams to ori-ent the viewer and display "real" dimensions of the imaged structures (Clarke and Dewhurst, 1996).

Thomas Willis (1621–1675) was a prominent scientist of brain anatomy in the 17th century. His work "Cerebri Anatome" provided a nearly complete account of the nervous system. Among his best-known contributions to the neurosciences are his pioneering work in the classification of the cranial nerves and the detailed de-scription and experimental analysis of the arterial circle (circulus arteriosus) at the base of the brain, commonly known today as the "Circle of Willis". Willis devel-oped the first alcohol fixative to preserve and harden the brain. The brain could then be easily removed intact from the skull, dissected, and sliced. Through this fixation process, Willis was able to describe (along with his illustrator, Christopher Wren) structures deep within the brain such as the corpus striatum. Prior to the fixation method, the brain tissue was flexible, and almost fluid and thus the structure bound-aries were difficult to visualize (Zimmer, 2004).

Charles Bell (1774–1842) was another crucial figure in imaging the brain be-fore the era of photography. Bell combined morphological studies with experiments and became one of the first neuroanatomists to distinguish sensory from motor nerves. It has been argued that Bell combined his skills as an anatomist and as an artist so successfully that his illustrations of the body were not only educational to anatomists but also aesthetically appealing. Accordingly, he was able to communi-cate images of the brain on a broad level and was well perceived by his contempo-raries (Gardner-Thorpe, 2004).

Even with all the above discussed developments in brain imaging, drawing techniques were not able to take the field further. The broader circulation of images required mass processing and distribution of the handmade drawings or paintings. The invention of printing techniques such as woodcuts, brought about the next step in the cascade of circulatory references. Woodcuts are limited, however, in their capability of displaying small structures in great detail. Accordingly, amplification of structures that were considered important and, reduction of less important structures was necessary in the transition step from drawings to woodcuts. The cascade can be displayed schematically as demonstrated in Figure 1. The cascade starts with the native brain, hidden in the skull, covered by layers of skin, bone, dura mater etc. The anatomist, through dissection must understand and reduce the complexity of the entire organ and amplify structures of interest. The artist – who may be the anatomist himself – then must convert the dissected organ into a two-dimensional drawing. The drawing is then engraved (or woodcut) and subsequently replicated through printing techniques. The next level of abstraction is thus initiated in the form of the printer, replication of the image and positioning the image in, for example, a book. Each reference step involves some reduction or amplification of elements existing in the prior step. In final form, the image is obviously different from the original brain from which it had been derived. Nonetheless, it is possible in theory to trace structures back to their origin. However, loss of information through amplification and reduction can make this objective difficult. In cases where a connection between a structure and the original object is not obvious per se, a reconstruction of the reference steps may facilitate the re-establishment of the link.

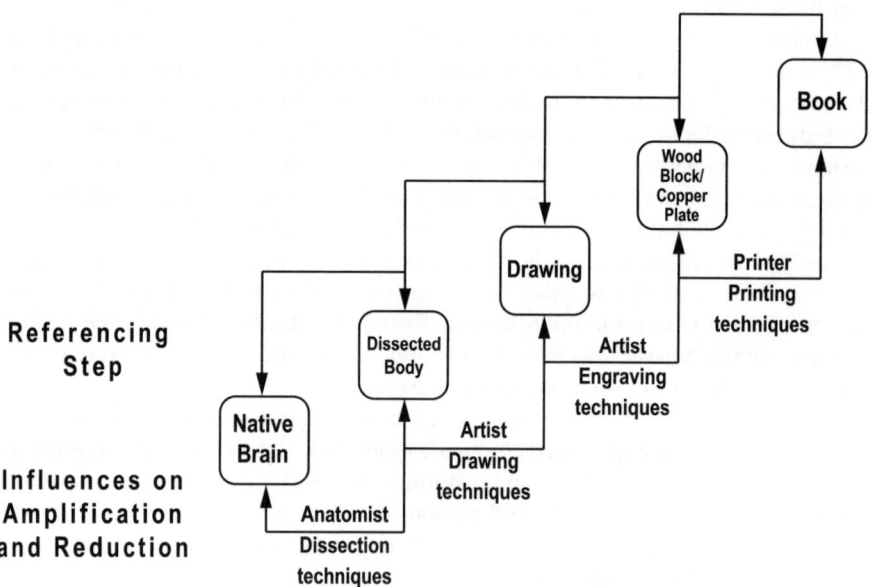

Figure 1: From brain to book.
Reference steps according to Latour's theory of circular references lead from the native brain to its abstraction depicted as an image in a book.

Transition 2: From Woodcuts to Radiographs

The discovery of the x-ray in 1895 by Wilhelm Konrad Röntgen (1845–1923) made it possible to visualize the internal environment of the living human body. The applicability of radiographs for medical purposes became immediately apparent. Depending on molecular composition, different tissues absorb x-rays to varying extents. The transmitted light causes a photoreaction on a photographic plate. The strength of this reaction depends on the amount of photons transmitted. Thus, the resulting grey-scale of the image represents a photon-count per unit, which can also be displayed numerically. In order to use the resulting images for clinical and scientific purposes it was necessary to establish certain standards concerning production and interpretation of radiographs.

Radiographs from skeletal structures or the lungs were comparably clear, while visualizing the human brain with the help of x-rays was at first difficult. Brain tissue (unlike other organs) was not displayed on the photo plates used. Manipulations were necessary to make brain structures visible. In 1918, Walter Dandy (1886–1946) developed "ventriculography" or "pneumencephalography", a technique by which air was pumped into the ventricles to replace the cerebrospinal fluid (Kilgore and Elster, 1995).[2] Through this method, images could be obtained that showed the ventricular structure of the brain in vivo. Pneumencephalograms followed the anatomical tradition of axial and frontal views. However, varying the position of the camera or the head allowed for the collection of information on the three-dimensional structure of the ventricles. Soon thereafter, in 1927, the Portuguese, Egas Moniz (1874–1955), introduced cerebral angiography (Eisenberg, 1992, pp. 323–346; Alper, 1999).

Crucial differences between radiographic images and drawings (that are ultimately printed) lie in the actors, systems, and techniques involved. Drawings result from visual perception, cognitive conversion, and artistic skills. Radiographs, on the contrary, are derived from "co-operation" of measurable physical phenomena: x-rays cause changes on photo plates that correspond to the density of tissue. Hence, radiographs are basically absorption pictures. Furthermore, radiography allows the creation of images in vivo, while anatomical drawings of the brain are composed from human corpses. Finally (and consequently), circulatory references differ substantially (Figure 2). First, dissection by an anatomist is not necessary with radiography. Instead, a physician applies contrast agents to visualize specific brain structures such as blood vessels. Subsequently, a technician (or the physician himself) generates x-rays with the help of electrodes and a diode and directs the x-rays to the brain. Through this technique a photo plate is imaged. The photo plate gives a representation of the brain that – during the next step of the cascade – must be made visible through chemical photo-development techniques. The end product is a new image of the brain that differs in production process and appearance from a drawing taken from a dissected body. As with a drawing, however, interpretation of the im-

---

2   On the ethical dimension of Dandy's innovation and his related dispute with Cushing see for example Pinkus (2001).

age must take into account the single steps of modulation, reduction, and amplification. For example, how and why a particular structure made visible by x-ray differs in appearance from the original tissue must be examined.

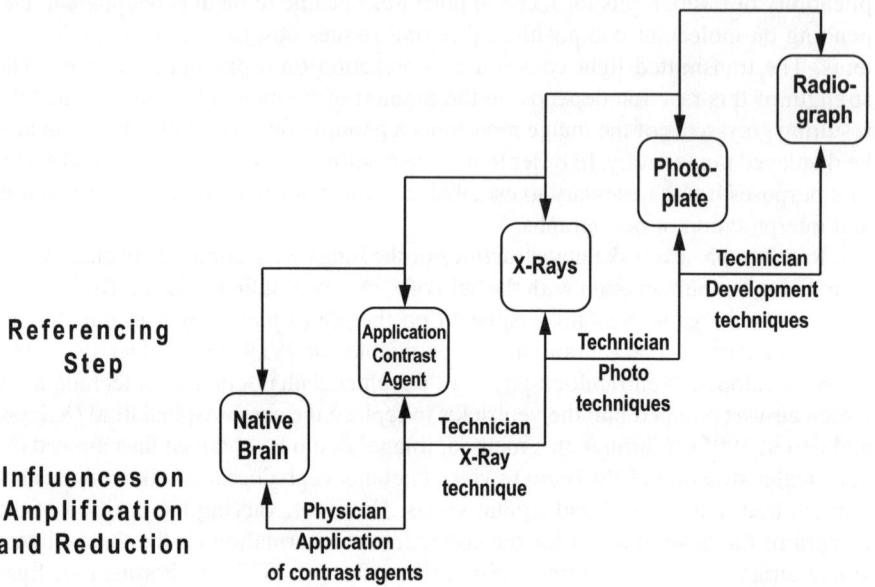

Figure 2: From brain to radiograph.
Reference steps according to Latour's theory of circular references lead from the native brain to its abstraction in an image depicted in a radiograph.

Transition 3: From Radiographs to Functional "Digital Imaging"

Structural "Digital Imaging"

With the advent of x-ray computed tomography (CT) in the 1970s and conventional magnetic resonance imaging (MRI) in the 1980s, studying brain structure in vivo became an important tool in clinical and scientific settings (Mazziotta, 2000). The introduction of these techniques represents the next step in the correlation of structural abnormalities and clinical symptoms.

In MRI, the signals of hydrogen nuclei are recorded. In the normal state atomic nuclei generate a magnetic moment. The axis of this magnetic moment is spinning with a specific frequency depending on the nuclei's particular properties as well as properties of the compound to which they belong and the environment. When placed in a magnetic field the spin vectors of such nuclei become aligned with the direction of the external field. With the application of a high-frequency electromagnetic impulse the spins rotate in-phase. After switching off the high-frequency impulse, the spins start to de-phase, and thus re-emit the energy that had been absorbed in the process of magnetization. This emission is then recorded. The localization of the source of the emission in three-dimensional space is thus made possible. On the basis of emission amplitude the source can be characterized and subsequently defined as specific tissues (such as cerebral white and grey matter, cerebrospinal fluid, bone etc.).

Through a stream of complex mathematical operations three-dimensional volumes can be generated through MRI. The resulting images consist of two-dimensional slices of the axial, coronal or sagittal plane. These data can then be used for structural analyses of both healthy and pathologically altered brains. Normal inter-subject variability of cerebral structures can be investigated (Tomaiuolo et al., 1999) and related to specific behavioural characteristics (Schlaug et al., 1995). In addition, MR-images can be analyzed in vertical and longitudinal studies of cerebral atrophy in specific degenerative diseases (e. g., Galton et al., 2001; Gorno-Tempini et al., 2004; Price et al., 2004; Studholme et al., 2004). Furthermore, structural brain images serve as a template for results of *functional* imaging studies, which will be described in the following section.

Functional "Digital Imaging"

According to an established model of cellular energy metabolism, there is evidence to suggest that cerebral activation is associated with an increase in energy metabolism evoking an increase in regional cerebral blood flow (rCBF). *Positron emission tomography* (PET) evaluates rCBF changes. Initially, *functional MRI* (fMRI) applied contrast agents to capture rCBF changes (e. g., Belliveau et al., 1991). Today, however, differences in magnetic susceptibility to deoxygenated and oxygenated hemoglobin are employed as an endogenous contrast agent to detect *blood oxygenation level dependent* (BOLD) changes (Ogawa et al., 1990; Raichle, 2001). The correlation of such changes with neuronal activity is still debated but there is ample evidence in favour of this hypothesis (e. g., Logothetis et al., 2001). Other means of measuring brain activity are *Electro-encephalography* (EEG), which records signals from large populations of cortical neurons via scalp electrodes, and *Magneto-encephalography* (MEG), which also registers electric potentials stemming from neuronal activity. These methods have very high temporal but comparably poor spatial resolution.

To visualize areas of rCBF or BOLD effect changes a series of complex mathematical operations must be performed. As shown in Figure 3, the first steps of the circular reference in producing an fMR-image include the application of a magnetic field and the subsequent recording of emitted energy. This step requires *pre-processing* which takes into account timing factors and subject movements. Pre-processing also transforms the individual data to align with a standard brain with a defined coordinate-set. After the pre-processing procedure, a *statistical analysis* is performed, resulting in "some index at each voxel of how the brain has responded to the experimental manipulations of interest" (Brett et al., 2002, p. 244). In the resulting "maps" that function as visual orientation guides, specific brain areas found to be involved in particular cognitive tasks are colour-coded. "Activation" is usually displayed in red to yellow tones while "deactivation" is generally represented with blue to green colours. Another popular depiction of the functioning brain is the so-called "glass brain view" provided by SPM (Statistical Parametric Mapping) software. The glass brain view provides an outline of the brain only, with no structural boundaries. In absence of the cerebral structures, "activated" areas have the appearance of solid structures with a grey scale encoding of statistic values. Averaging of individual subject data enables the demonstration of group effects.

The next step in brain analysis is "activation labelling". This step faces several problems (Brett et al., 2002). First, labelling must be adapted to coordinates, macroanatomy, or microanatomy. Spatially normalized data are arranged in a stereotaxic space (Talairach and Tournoux, 1988) so that single points of space can be described by three coordinates (x, y, z) to enable inter-subject and even inter-species comparisons. Nonetheless, coordinate labelling has its limitations due to methodological variability (Brett et al., 2002). Despite spatial normalization of individual data, inter-subject macroanatomical (e. g., Tomaiuolo et al., 1999) as well as microanatomical (e. g., Amunts et al., 1999) variability presents problems. Furthermore, it is not possible to infer cytoarchitectural boundaries (Brodmann areas) from macroanatomical landmarks such as gyri or sulci. This inter-individual variability in gross anatomy and cytoarchitecture has been demonstrated in detail with regard to several brain regions (Hasnain et al., 1998; Amunts et al., 1999; Tomaiuolo et al., 1999; Rademacher et al., 2001; Rademacher et al., 2002; Amunts et al., 2005).

In summary, functional "digital images" are the result of two chains of transformative steps. Both chains involve the measurement of nuclear characteristics of tissues and the collection of binary data. The creation of statistical maps requires the alignment of structural and functional data to project functional results onto a structural matrix. This step, as indicated in Figure 3, can be considered a converging step resulting in the visualization of the generated data. In this way, both chains of references as well as their shared steps differ substantially from those of drawings or radiographs. The images created by these techniques are *primarily* data-driven. Unlike other brain imaging techniques that transform information into binary data *after* the creation of the image, the collection of binary data is one of the first crucial steps in the process of digital imaging production. However, similar to drawings, digital images are based on a large amount of data and are prone to manipulations such as the amplification or reduction of signals causing a distortion of the image from the original organ.[3] Contrary to drawings or radiographs the amplifications or reductions in each transformation step cannot be detected in fMRIs. Paradoxically, fMRIs seems to offer an objective view of the brain. The fMR-image does not present itself as data but as a picture of reality. The French philosopher Jean Baudrillard introduced the term "simulacrum" to describe such a paradox. "Simulacrum" refers to the loss of the original picture (or at least the reference) and its replacement by the simulation of a representation (Baudrillard, 1978, pp. 14

---

3   In contrast to the artificial elements inherent in the process of producing fMRI images the expression "artifacts" in this context is not used to name the resulting image but the disturbing factors inherent in the process of producing such images ("noise"; "motion artifacts" etc.).

sqq.). Even the conventional and culturally bound "activation" or "deactivation" colour-codes contribute to this impression. These simulations enhance the original impact of the image and are often (mis-) taken as intrinsic characteristics of the original tissue (Gombrich, 1978, p. 14). As a consequence, amateur spectators may consider them to be more real than their natural counterparts according to a "principle of disjunction inherent to scientific depictions" (Bredekamp and Werner, 2003, p. 15).

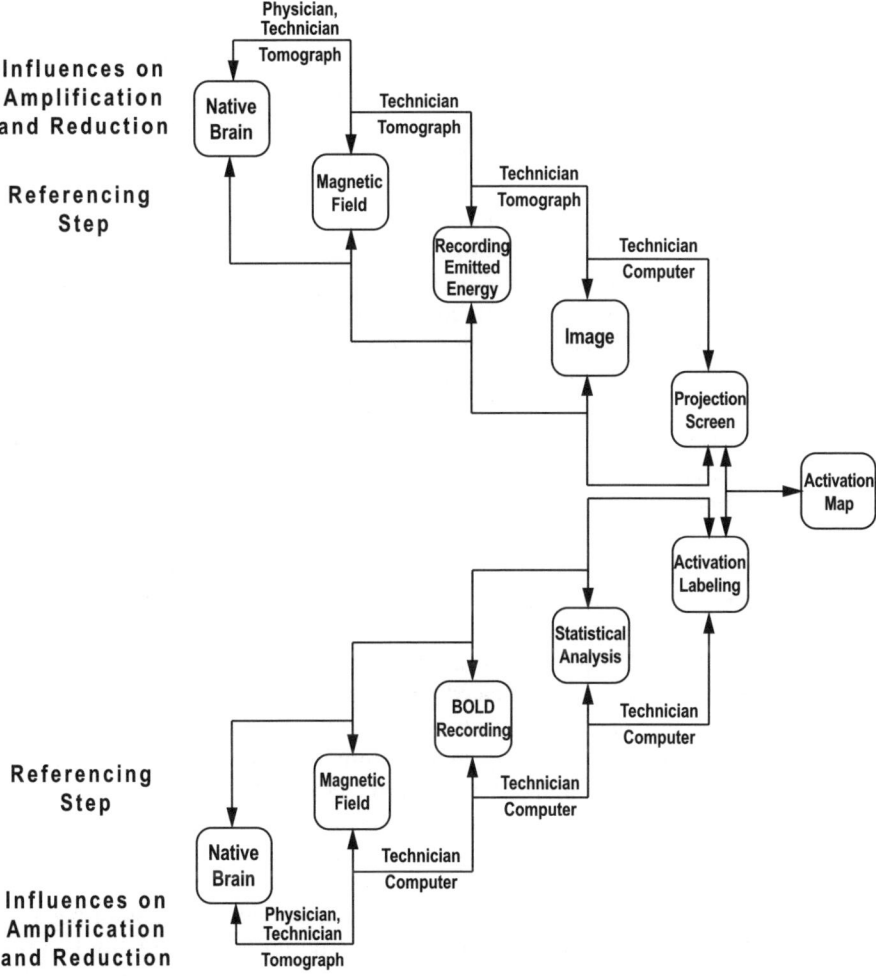

Figure 3: From brain to activation map.
Reference steps according to Latour's theory of circular references lead from the native brain to its abstraction in the form of an activation map. The single steps are described in the text.

PERSPECTIVES

We schematically examined the production process of brain images under the framework of "circulatory references" for three epochs, which can be very roughly classified as pre-modernistic, modernistic and post-modernistic approaches. Methods of amplifying and reducing information and the intent of the images differ substantially. Imaging the brain includes imagination (imagining the brain) which is dependent on education and conceptual constraints. In addition, from a historical perspective the three methods represent steps on the way from the visualization to the virtualization of brain structure and function. "Virtualization" indicates the creation of a virtual reality, the creation of a simulation of a brain with the help of computing techniques. While drawings, woodcuts and radiographs are produced by artisan skills or physical phenomena alone, digital images are ultimately the result of computing technology. "Digital images" provide a new way of abstracting information from the brain.

Drawings from the pre-modern era were produced by artists or artistically trained anatomists. The main purpose of these drawings was to illustrate anatomical findings and theories leading to symbolic, more diagrammatic images, and to a morphological emphasis of certain structures. Elements considered "important" by the producer were highlighted while those deemed insignificant were minimized. "Form", not "function" dominated the image. Radiographs from the modern era served mostly as a diagnostic tool. Their interpretation is fit into common schools of reasoning, "Denkstile" as Fleck named them (e. g. pneumencephalographs).[4] In addition, radiographs gave a more objective view of the brain (by using seemingly undeceivable photographing techniques) compared to subjective interpretations of visual perceptions inherent to drawings. As a result, a higher epistemic value was attributed to radiographs than to drawings. Finally, whereas drawings represented an abstraction from a number of brains, radiographs initially were related specifically to one particular individual. The imaging of "form", not "function" (as with drawing in the pre-modernist era) was the main focus.

Since the 1970s, more sophisticated technical devices such as CT scans have allowed for more precise correlations between clinical observations and structural abnormalities of brain tissue. Finally, in the postmodern era "digital imaging" has merged diagnostic and illustrative rationales for producing images. While radiographic techniques are still physical and thus considered objective, the visualization technique in functional neuroimaging is a) genuinely digital and b) heavily dependent on the image producer's influence (similar to drawings). Furthermore, in order to conduct group studies, brain images taken from an individual are conformed to a standardized template. The resulting brain images do not exist in reality and the resulting activation maps display virtual *representations* of cerebral functions. The spectator of neuroimages relies on the final product, which is quasi-automatically generated. A variety of factors contribute to the acceptance of the resulting images.

---

4   See the paper by Friedrich in this volume.

The spectator generally does not reflect on the production process behind functional "digital images"" while accepting their outcome. This has an impact on the epistemological value of the images. The epistemic status of those images can be considered as two-fold. On the one hand they serve as illustrations for theories on brain function. On the other hand they are also the source of new theories. Spectators must be aware, however, that these images are the result of a long chain of computing steps influenced by the scientist. In a way, the scientist becomes an artist comparable to the pre-modernist illustrator. In terms of the history of art, the scientist is "making" an object by preparation, colourization and exposing. This production process allows for adjustment to the final result. The resulting brain images follow stylistic traditions set in anatomical drawings. Spectators are familiar with the proposed visualizations and thus accept them as "real". A digitally produced image of the brain is less a realistic account of the physical brain and more a visualization of numbers translated into signs supported by a technical epistemic framework. And as with any media: the process of encoding is deeply connected with the spectator's competence for reading (decoding) and comprehending.

Reading and comprehending capabilities are often enhanced by "special" effects. Three dimensional perspective, rotating images, shadow and colour effects lead to "hyper-realistic" representations. In his theory on contemporary culture, Baudrillard expressed the opinion that "the hyperreal itself [...] retains all the features, the whole discourse of traditional production, but it is no longer anything but its scaled-down refraction [...]. Thus everywhere the hyperrealism of simulation is translated by the hallucinatory resemblance of the real to itself" (Baudrillard, 1993, p. 23). This, of course, is a conclusion that holds true for imaging and imagining the brain with the help of functional digital methods. While the beauty of produced images may lead to an unquestioned acceptance by the layman, the ambiguity of the heuristic value needs to be clarified by the scientist.

REFERENCES

Alper, M.G., 1999. Three pioneers in the early history of neuroradiology: the Snyder lecture. Doc. Ophthalmol. 98, 29–49.

Amunts, K., Kedo, O., Kindler, M., et al., 2005. Cytoarchitectonic mapping of the human amygdala, hippocampal region and entorhinal cortex: intersubject variability and probability maps. Anat. Embryol. (Berl.). 210(5–6), 343–352.

Amunts, K., Schleicher, A., Burgel, U., et al. 1999. Broca's region revisited: cytoarchitecture and intersubject variability. J. Comp. Neurol. 412(2), 319–341.

Baudrillard, J., 1978. Agonie des Realen. Merve-Verlag, Berlin.

Baudrillard, J., 1995. Simulacra and Simulation. University of Michigan Press, Michigan.

Bechtel, W., 2000. From imaging to believing: epistemic issues in generating biological data, in: Bechtel, W. (Ed.), Biology and Epistemology. Cambridge University Press, Cambridge, pp. 138–163.

Belliveau, J.W., Kennedy, D.N., Jr., McKinstry, R.C., et al., 1991. Functional mapping of the human visual cortex by magnetic resonance imaging. Science. 254(5032), 716–719.

Bredekamp, H., Werner, G. (Eds.), 2003. Bildwelten des Wissens. Kunsthistorisches Jahrbuch für Bildkritik. Akademie Verlag, Berlin.

Breidbach, O., 1997. Die Materialisierung des Ichs: Zur Geschichte der Hirnforschung im 19. und 20. Jahrhundert. Suhrkamp, Frankfurt.

Brett, M., Johnsrude, I. S. and Owen, A. M., 2002. The problem of functional localization in the human brain. Nat. Rev. Neurosci. 3(3), 243–249.

Clarke, E., Dewhurst, K. (Eds.), 1996. An illustrated history of brain function. Imaging the brain from antiquity to the present. Norman Publishing, San Francisco.

Eisenberg, R. L., 1992. Radiology. An illustrated history. Mosby, St. Louis.

Fleck, L., 1983 (1947). Schauen, sehen, wissen, in: Fleck L. (Ed.), Ludwik Fleck. Erfahrung und Tatsache. Gesammelte Aufsätze. Suhrkamp, Frankfurt, pp. 147–174.

Galton, C. J., Gomez-Anson, B., Antoun, N., et al., 2001. Temporal lobe rating scale: application to Alzheimer's disease and frontotemporal dementia. J. Neurol. Neurosurg. Psychiatry 70(2), 165–173.

Gardner-Thorpe, C., 2004. The Art of Sir Charles Bell, in: Clifford Rose, F. (Ed.), Neurology of the Arts: Painting, Music, Literature. Imperial College Press, London, pp. 99–128.

Gombrich, E. H., 1978. Meditations on a Hobby Horse. Phaidon, London.

Gombrich, E. H., 1987. Zur Kunst der Renaissance. Vol. 3: Die Entdeckung des Sichtbaren. Klett-Cotta, Stuttgart.

Gorno-Tempini, M. L., Dronkers, N. F., Rankin, K. P., et al., 2004. Cognition and anatomy in three variants of primary progressive aphasia. Ann. Neurol. 55(3), 335–346.

Hagner, M., 1997. Homo cerebralis. Der Wandel vom Seelenorgan zum Gehirn. Wissenschaftliche Buchgesellschaft, Darmstadt.

Hasnain, M. K., Fox, P. T., Woldorff, M. G., 1998. Intersubject variability of functional areas in the human visual cortex. Hum. Brain Mapp. 6(4), 301–315.

Illes, J., Racine, E., 2005. Imaging or Imagining? A Neuroethics Challenge Informed by Genetics. Am. J. Bioeth. 5(2), 5–18

Kilgore, E. J., Elster, A. D., 1995. Walter Dandy and the history of ventriculography. Radiology. 194(3), 657–660.

Lantos, P. L., 1983. Changing images of the brain. Psychol. Med. 13(2), 255–266.

Latour, B., 1999. Pandora's hope: essays on the reality of science studies. Harvard University Press, Cambridge, Mass.

Linden, D. E., 2002. Five hundred years of brain images. Arch. Neurol. 59(2), 308–313.

Logothetis, N. K., Pauls, J., Augath, M., et al., 2001. Neurophysiological investigation of the basis of the fMRI signal. Nature. 412(6843), 150–157.

Maudgil, D. D., 1997. Changing interpretations of the human cortical pattern. Arch. Neurol. 54(6), 769–775.

Mazziotta, J. C., 2000. Imaging: window on the brain. Arch. Neurol. 57(10), 1413–1421.

Meyer, A., 1971. Historical aspects of cerebral anatomy. Oxford University Press, London.

Mitchell, W. J. T.: 1986, Iconology: image, text, ideology. Chicago: University of Chicago Press.

Mitchell, W. J. T., 1994. The Pictorial Turn, in: Mitchell, W. J. T. (Ed.), Picture Theory. Essays on Verbal and Visual Representation. University of Chicago Press, Chicago, pp. 11–34.

Ogawa, S., Lee, T. M., Kay, A. R., et al., 1990. Brain magnetic resonance imaging with contrast dependent on blood oxygenation. Proceedings of the National Academy of Sciences 87(24), 9868–9872.

Panofsky, E., 1985. Die Perspektive als "symbolische Form", in: Panofsky, E. (Ed.), Aufsätze zu Grundfragen der Kunstwissenschaft. Hrsg. v. H. Oberer und E. Verheyen. Spiess, Berlin, pp. 99–167.

Pinkus, R. L., 2001. Mistakes as a Social Construct: An Historical Approach. Kennedy Institute of Ethics Journal 11(2), 117–133.

Price, S., Paviour, D., Scahill, R., et al., 2004. Voxel-based morphometry detects patterns of atrophy that help differentiate progressive supranuclear palsy and Parkinson's disease. Neuroimage. 23(2), 663–669.

Rademacher, J., Burgel, U., Geyer, S., et al., 2001. Variability and asymmetry in the human precentral motor system. A cytoarchitectonic and myeloarchitectonic brain mapping study. Brain. 124(Pt 11), 2232–2258.

Rademacher, J., Burgel, U., Zilles, K., 2002. Stereotaxic localization, intersubject variability, and interhemispheric differences of the human auditory thalamocortical system. Neuroimage. 17(1), 142–160.

Raichle, M. E., 2001. Cognitive neuroscience. Bold insights. Nature. 412(6843), 128–130.

Roeck, B., 2003. Visual turn? Kulturgeschichte und die Bilder. Geschichte und Gesellschaft 29, 294–315.

Rorty, R., 1967. The linguistic turn: Recent essays in Philosophical method. University of Chicago Press, Chicago.

Saunders J. B., O'Malley C. D., 1982. The anatomical drawings of Andreas Vesalius. Bonanza Books, New York.

Sawday, J., 1995. The body emblazoned: dissection and the human body in Renaissance culture. Routledge, London.

Schlaug, G., Jäncke, L., Huang, Y., Steinmetz, H., 1995. In vivo evidence of structural brain asymmetries in musicians. Science 267(5198), 699–701.

Schott, G. D., 2000. Illustrating cerebral function: the iconography of arrows. Philos. Trans. R. Soc. Lond. B Biol. Sci. 355(1404), 1789–1799.

Studholme, C., Cardenas, V., Blumenfeld, R., et al.: 2004, Deformation tensor morphometry of semantic dementia with quantitative validation. Neuroimage 21(4), 1387–1398.

Talairach, J., Tournoux, P., 1988. Co-planar stereotaxic atlas of the human brain. Thieme, Stuttgart.

Tessman, P. A., Suarez, J. I., 2002. Influence of early printmaking on the development of neuroanatomy and neurology. Arch. Neurol. 59(12), 1964–1969.

Tomaiuolo, F., MacDonald, J. D., Caramanos, Z., et al., 1999. Morphology, morphometry and probability mapping of the pars opercularis of the inferior frontal gyrus: an in vivo MRI analysis. Eur. J. Neurosci. 11(9), 3033–3046.

Tsafrir, J., Ohry, A., 2001. Medical illustration: from caves to cyberspace. Health Info. Libr. J. 18(2), 99–109.

Zimmer, C., 2004. Soul Made Flesh: The Discovery of the Brain and How it Changed the World. Free Press, New York.

III. IMAGING THE BODY – PRACTICES AND MEDIA

ICONOGRAPHY AND WAX MODELS
IN ITALIAN EARLY SMALLPOX VACCINATION[1]

Fabio Zampieri, Alberto Zanatta, Maurizio Rippa Bonati

INTRODUCTION

Luigi Sacco (1769–1863) was the main protagonist of the early vaccination campaign in Italy. He found a native source of vaccine lymph, with which he personally vaccinated more than 500,000 people and furnished all of Italy and some countries in the Middle East. Starting from the pictures of his books, Sacco proposed to create wax models of *real* and *spurious* smallpox pustules in human, cow, sheep and horse.

At this time anatomical ceroplastic was a technique already well established in many medical centres. It was related to the necessity to faithfully reproduce the parts of human anatomy for didactic and researches purposes. This necessity started to be appreciated from the rediscovery of human anatomy during the Renaissance and the successive comprehension of its importance in medical practice. The reproduction by wax models of human and animal parts was preceded by the method of injection established during the early XVII Century, through which an organ was injected with a mixture of wax and other chemicals for its preservation. Jan Swammerdam (1637–1680) and Frederik Ruysch (1638–1731) has been the early most famous producers of these injected preparations. Another early technique used for the preservations of human organs and bodies for medical purposed has been the mummification. Nevertheless both these techniques soon revealed their limits, because the preparations quickly deteriorated with use and, at any case, they didn't preserve with precision the three-dimensional structure of the organ. Injection, for instance, was suitable for showing the vascular tree of parenchymal organs, but does not allow the faithful reproduction of the whole organ structure (Maraldi et al. 2000, p. 9). From the development of waxwork modelling during the Renaissance for artistic purposes, anatomical ceroplastic originated around the second half of the XVII Century (see the two volumes of the Congress on "Wax Modelling in Art and Science": AAVV 1977) and soon became widely used and appreciated. Italy has been the country in which this new technique originated, particularly in the schools of Bologna and Florence, and where it finds its maximal development. If the first anatomical ceroplastic was more concerned with the aesthetic of representation rather than the precision of anatomical details, the successive phase at the core of the XVIII Century was deeply concerned with the naturalistic reproduction of the normal anatomy of human body and organs, while the last period of ceroplastic, between the end of XVIII Century and the whole XIX Century, has been character-

---

1   A previous version of this text has been published in the journal Medicine Studies.

ized by the representation of pathological anatomy (Pirson 2009). The wax works related to smallpox and vaccine belong to this last phase.

The purpose of the wax models inspired by the picture of the Luigi Sacco's books, which are the object of this text, was to permit the identification, by doctors and all other health operators, of the correct pustules from which to extract active lymph for vaccination. The Museum of Pathological Anatomy of the Padua University Medical School owns four anatomical waxes that correspond exactly to the explicative pictures in Sacco's 1809 treatise on vaccines. These same models are also found at the University of Milan, Pavia, and Bologna – the main cities of the "Cisalpine Republic", the state of North Italy formed during Sacco's time after the Napoleon conquest.

We believe that the history of the diffusion of these models can be paradigmatic to characterize the birth of contemporary medicine, in which images and virtual models serve as fundamental didactic and diagnostic tools. Contemporary medicine developed mainly by the imposition of three disciplines in the course of XIX Century: experimental physiology, pathological anatomy and microbiology. Pathological anatomy was based on the idea that structural lesion was the ultimate reference of the specificity of each disease. Microbiology stated that each infectious disease was caused by a specific microscopic living entity. Living entities which could be identified by their specific microscopic morphologies. In both these cases, the determination of the disease specificity was related to a structural and localistic perspective. We can say that the diffusion of images and wax models about vaccination in the early XIX Century could be seen as a prelude of the fully development of pathological anatomy and microbiological perspective in the following course of the century. Images and wax models represented the seat and structure of smallpox and vaccine pustules. The intention of the promoters of these tools was to show the difference between smallpox and vaccine. A difference which was characterized by the structural and chromatic properties of the pustules. It is clear that in this operation was already effective the idea of the strict relationship between specificity of the diseases and its morphological manifestation.

EARLY ICONOGRAPHY ABOUT VACCINATION

The wide use of iconography about smallpox only started with the advent of vaccination, discovered by Edward Jenner (1749–1823), physician and surgeon of Gloucester and scholar of John Hunter (1728–1793) (Wilkenstein, 1992). Vaccination against smallpox was first practiced by inoculating humans with lymph from the pustules of cowpox, a similar disease that affected the bovine nipple and was able to induce immunity against smallpox in humans. Jenner based his discovery on the observation (supported by popular tradition) that the cowpox-infected milkmaids of his country were protected against smallpox.

Although Jenner never published images of cowpox, he provided the first images of human pustules induced by vaccination. In his first treatise on vaccination, he published a coloured engraving of a pustule in the hand of dairymaid Sarah Nelmens (see Fig. 1). Jenner felt the necessity to visualize the most typical vaccine

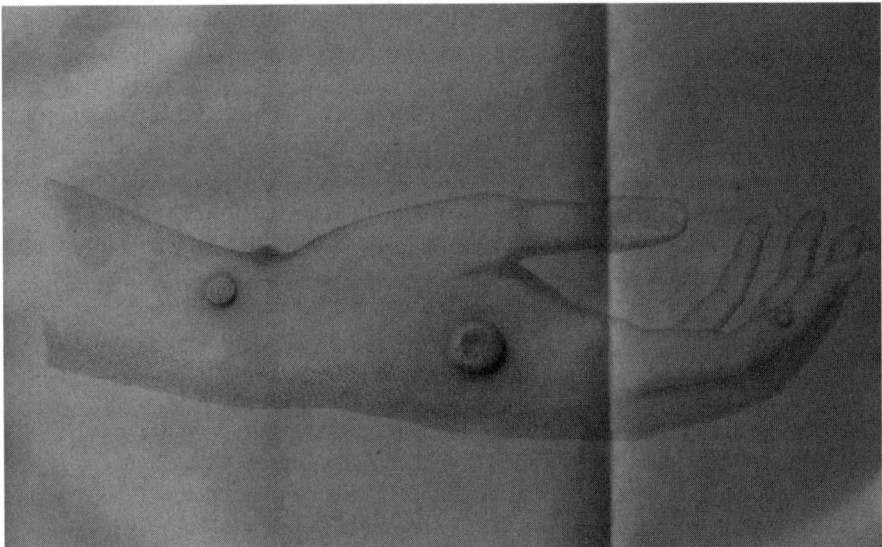

Fig. 1: Jenner's first image of vaccine pustules

pustule to show its structural and chromatic specificity (Jenner, 1798, p. 31). This publication by Jenner provides the introduction of the variable *space* – by the representation of the structure and colour of the pustule – in the scientific discourse about smallpox. This variable was used by Jenner to acquaint readers with the differences between the pustules of smallpox and vaccine. He published two additional plates about vaccine pustules that were quite similar to the typical pustule of smallpox: one for an areola around the eruption (Jenner, 1798, p. 38) and one for the emergence of some minor pustules around the main one (Jenner, 1798, p. 40).

Jenner had two purposes for his images of the vaccine pustules. The similitude between the vaccine and smallpox pustules was ultimately an indirect proof of the efficacy of the vaccine. The images also showed that the vaccine pustule was different from that of smallpox, particularly in terms of its milder effects and healthier evolution; this fact also was an indirect proof that the vaccine was less dangerous than inoculation. These ideas became more evident and explicit in the successive iconographical representations of vaccine.

In 1799, one year after the publication of his first *Inquiry*, Jenner published the *Further Observations on the Variolae Vaccinae* that treated the fundamental question of the *spurious vaccine*. The theme of the spurious vaccine was predominant in the 19th discussion about the new practice. Some physicians observed that the lymph extracted from cow or from vaccine human pustules was not always effective in inducing immunity in their patients. This fact was obviously of primary importance, because it could discredit the new practice (Jenner, 1799, p. 1). Jenner carefully analyzed several reasons for the production of this spurious vaccine (Jenner, 1799, p. 4). Strangely, Jenner did not think it was important to visualise the spurious cow pustules (those in which the lymph had "suffered a decomposition", for instance, or was ulcerated).

In 1800 Jenner published *A Continuation of Facts and Observations Relative to the Variolae Vaccine or Cow Pox* (Jenner 1800) and the second edition of his *Inquiry* (Jenner 1800a). In *Continuation*, Jenner criticized the results of William Woodville (1752–1805), physician of the "Hospital for Small-pox and Inoculation" of London (Jenner 1800, pp. 7–8). Woodville had found that vaccinated people sometimes could furnish ineffective lymph to vaccinate other patients. He soon recognized that good lymph was extracted in the mildest pustules and in the period of their maximal maturation, but not before or after (Woodville 1799, in McVail 1896: 1273).

The discussions between Jenner and Woodville led to an anonymous publication in 1800 that probably was edited by Jenner and Woodville themselves: *A Comparative Statement of Facts and Observations Relative to the Cow-Pox* (Anonymous, 1800). This publication provides the first comparison between images of the vaccine and smallpox pustules. It also provides the first plate that visualises, by a sequence of images, the evolution of both pustules (see Fig. 2). The anonymous author (1800) wrote:

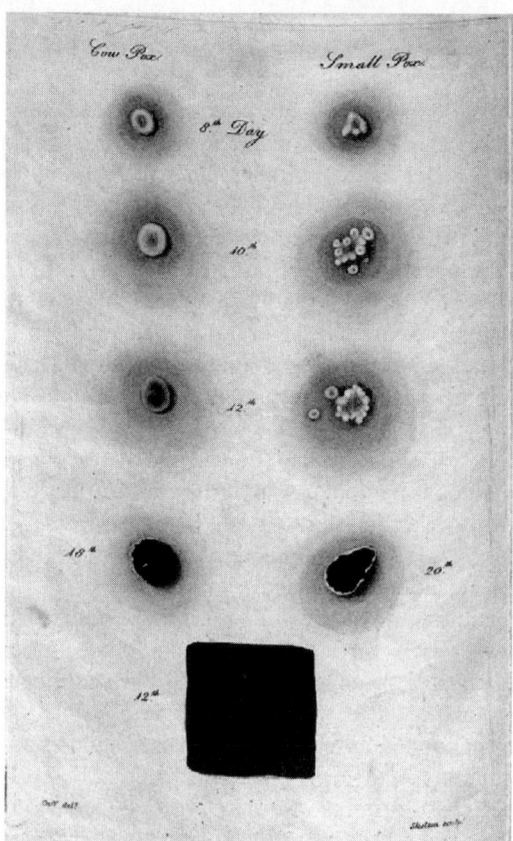

Fig. 2: comparative visualisation of vaccine and smallpox pustules

Those who engage in vaccine inoculation ought to be aware that they cannot be too cautious in the choice of the virus, or too attentive to its local action. If the virus be taken without discrimination, the operator will be subject to the errors which may have already committed. [...] Perhaps the benevolent views of those who may be anxious to shield their domestics, and the laborious poor, form the dire effects of the Small-Pox, cannot be more effectually promoted than by contrasting the varioulous and vaccine pustules at different periods of their progress. For this purpose the annexed plate was prepared, in which the pustules are delineated and coloured from nature (pp. 39–40).

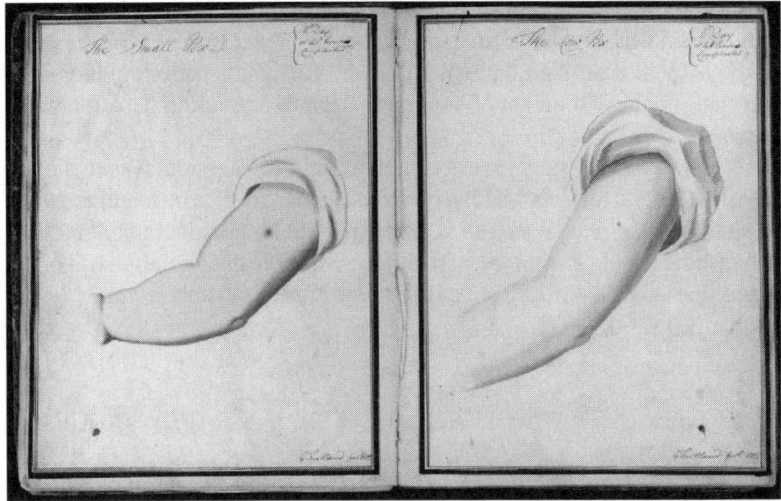

Fig. 3: first day of vaccine and smallpox pustules

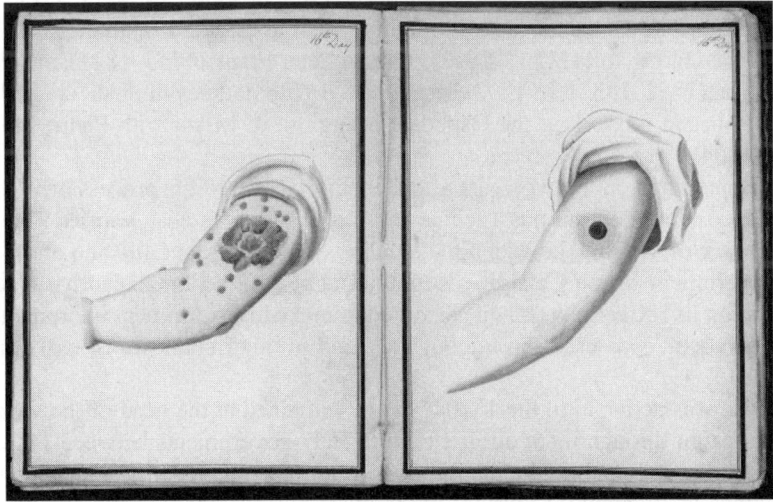

Fig. 4: 16th day of vaccine and smallpox pustules

With this plate, beside the variable *space*, the second fundamental variable *time* entered the discussion for the first time. Time corresponds to the visualisation of different stages of the evolution of vaccine and smallpox pustules.

An early example of the "philosophy of visualisation" was published in 1802 by George Kirtland (1753–1837). This example is probably the best among the plates published in England, French, Germany, and Italy in the first years of the 19th century (McVail, 1896, pp. 1276–7). There were 30 plates showing two arms each, one with a vaccine pustule and the other with a smallpox pustule, from the first day of infection through the 16th day (Figs. 3 and 4). These tables were reproduced in a special issue of *The British Medical Journal* of 1896 for the Jennerian Centenary. McVail described them as follows: "Kirtland's plates are themselves so eloquent that it is almost an act of supererogation to attempt to describe what is so well depicted" (McVail 1896: 1276).

The effect, when the pages were turned in rapid succession, was that of an animation in which pustules gradually evolved in their different manifestations. Although similar, vaccine and smallpox have specific and distinct phenomenologies, and the vaccine displays a more beneficial evolution than smallpox. This fact is something that only a similar series of images could transmit so immediately and unequivocally.

ICONOGRAPHY AND WAX MODELS IN ITALIAN EARLY VACCINATION

Luigi Sacco, also called The Italian Jenner (Biagini 1808) and The Apostle of Vaccination (Freschi, 1851, p. 105), was the major protagonist of the first vaccination campaign in North Italy. Sacco was born in Varese on 9 March 1769 in a modest but well-off family. After his studies in grammar and rhetoric, he moved to Milan at age 17 and then to the University of Pavia. He studied philosophy, natural sciences, and medicine, and he contacted with luminaries such as Lazzaro Spallanzani (1729–1799), Alessandro Volta (1745–1827), Johann Peter Frank (1745–1821), and Antonio Scarpa (1752–1832). In 1792, he graduated with degrees in medicine and surgery and began to work at the Ospedale Maggiore of Milan with Pietro Moscati (1739–1824).

In September, 1800, two years after Jenner discovered the process of vaccination, Sacco identified the pus vaccine in a group of cows near Varese. With this local source of vaccine, he ended the smallpox epidemics in Giussano and Sesto. The government of the Cisalpine Republic named Sacco the executive chief of vaccination in 1801. He was then permitted to make his experiment in orphanages. Sacco's vaccine was used throughout Italy and in other countries of east Europe and Asia.

Sacco was active until the 1820s, and he remained at the head of the vaccination campaign through three different North Italy governments between 1801 and 1809 – Cisalpine Republic, Italian Republic, and Italian Kingdom – which included the regions of Piemonte, Liguria, Lombardia, Emilia Romagna, and Veneto. The cities of Bologna and Brescia gave Sacco gold medals for his successful elimination of the smallpox epidemic. The city of Milan dedicated a monument to him on 29 April, 1858, which is still visible in the Ospedale Maggiore (Ferrario, 1858).

In 1801, Sacco published his first book on vaccination, entitled *Practical Observation on the Use of Cow-pox for Preserving against Small-pox* (hereafter referred to as *Observation*; Sacco, 1801). Sacco reported his discovery of vaccine lymph in Italian cows, from which he was able to inoculate first himself and then 300 patients. Their cases are described in the book (Sacco, 1801, pp. 60–158). He also made some interesting observations. To prove that the lymph from the pustules of cows was the original source of the vaccine "germ", he reintroduced vaccine lymph from human pustules to the cow nipple. As a result, he observed the emergence of the same pustules (Sacco, 1801, pp. 202–3). Table I at the end of the book displays cows' nipples infected by spontaneous or induced pustules (see Fig. 5). Table II shows two instruments for vaccination and a series of images representing the evolution of human vaccine pustules (see Fig. 6). The purpose of this visualisation was clearly stated by Sacco:

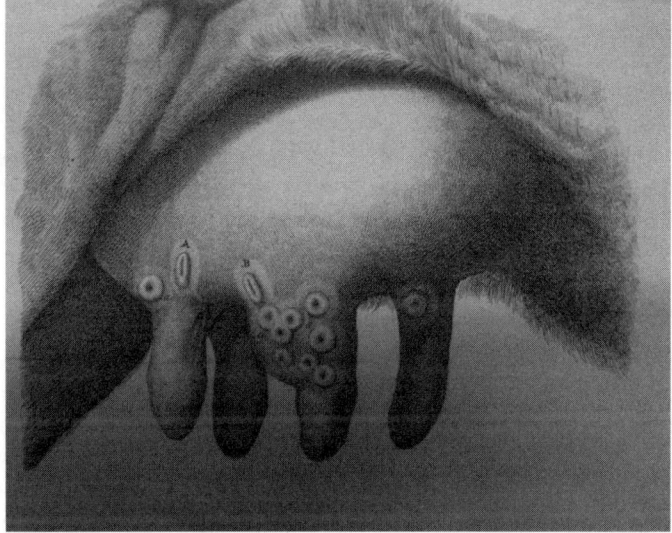

Fig. 5: spontaneous (a) and induced (A, B) cow pox pustules

The real vaccine absolutely has not to be confused with the spurious one. It should be a fatal error to consider that the second has the same effect of the first. The real preserve to human smallpox, while the second didn't do that. Both these diseases have distinct characters and I'll never stop to repeat that it is of the maximal importance to be able to recognise them even at the first sight, which is possible only after several experiences, errors and observations (Sacco, 1801, pp. 193–4).

Sacco published a second monograph about vaccination in 1803, entitled *Memory on the Vaccine as Unique Method to Extirpate Smallpox Radically, Directed to the Governments which Love the Prosperity of Their Nations* (hereafter referred to as

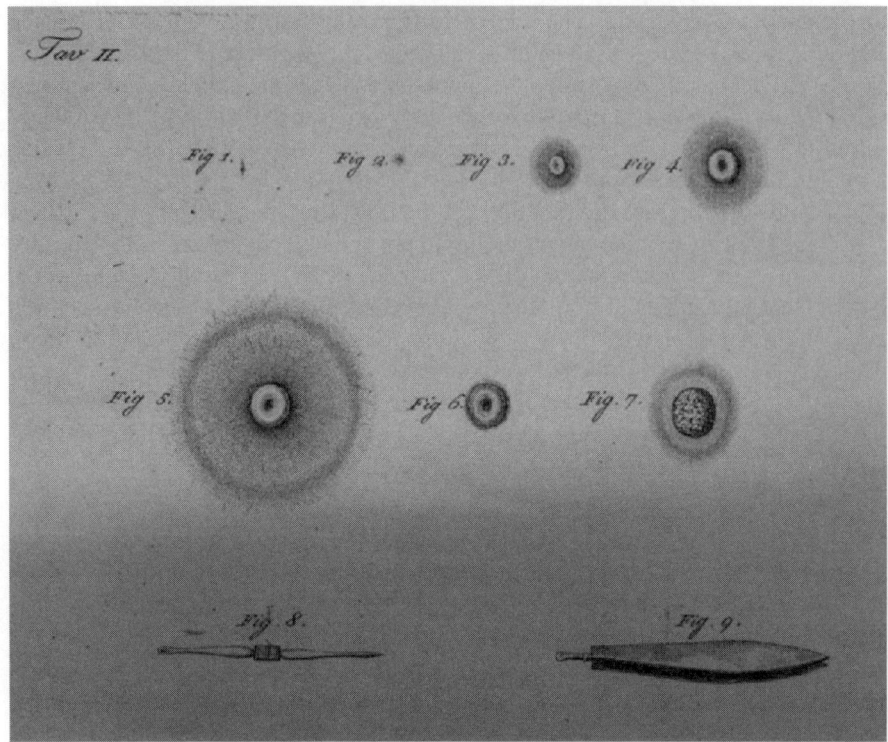

Fig. 6: evolution of human vaccine pustule and instrument for vaccination

Memory; Sacco, 1803). Inspired by this book, Prussia, Bavaria, and some other Italian Districts, such as Parma, Lucca, and Tuscan, adopted the vaccination laws of the Italian Republic (Ferrario, 1858a, p. 26). Although this book does not contain any images, it does offer a fundamental quotation for understanding the successive iconographical and wax models productions inspired by Sacco. He asserted that midwifes should be instructed in the vaccination procedure, so that they could learn to distinguish real from spurious pustules:

> To fix the attention of the population, and, particularly, of physicians, surgeons and midwifes, and to avoid the danger of reaching doubtful or misleading results, it should be prepared tables with well coloured drawings or, even better, two arms made by wax, one with pustules of real vaccine, another with spurious and anomalous pustules. Those pictures should be multiplied and send to every chief town for being regularly examined by professors and midwifes. (Sacco, 1803, p. 36)

This statement demonstrates the importance that Sacco gave to images and three-dimensional wax models. He advised the local administrations to create wax models for popular diffusion and for physicians, surgeons, and midwifes.

In 1809, Sacco published his masterpiece, *The Treatise of Vaccination with Observations on Grease and Sheep-pox* (hereafter referred to as *Treatise*; Sacco,

1809), in which he published those "well-coloured drawings" that he retained as the best way to spread the necessary knowledge about the practice of vaccination. This book was a massive monograph in which he described the practice and several experiences of vaccination in 14 chapters and 224 pages. He instructed that the lymph for vaccination could be obtained mainly from cowpox, but also from similar diseases in horse (*grease*) and sheep (*sheep-pox*) (Sacco, 1809, p. 8).

Sacco addressed the nature of the disease, refuting the common hypothesis that smallpox was a spontaneous, internal disease caused by a "putrefaction" of humours. He supported that it was an infectious disease transmitted by the eggs of microscopic insects, which could live outside the host organisms in a state of "apparent dead" and spread through the atmosphere (Sacco, 1809, pp. 21–3). He dedicated an entire chapter to some human "cutaneous expulsions" that were similar, but etiologically different, to smallpox (e. g., chicken-pox, scarlet fever, rubella, and others) (Sacco, 1809, pp. 155–166). He analyzed the "influence of vaccination on the augmentation of population" (Sacco, 1809, pp. 167–71), described experimentations of the vaccine inoculation of other animals (dog, pig, and others) (Sacco, 1809, pp. 172–8), and reported microscopic observations and chemical manipulations of the vaccine lymph (Sacco, 1809, pp. 179–90).

The principal question addressed by Sacco was how and from where to extract good lymph for obtaining a true vaccination and not a spurious one. Sacco maintained that it was important to recognize the real pustule from the spurious; the most essential, consistent, and characteristic symptoms were circumscribed only to the pustule, while the others where more fluctuant (Sacco, 1809, p. 45).

The spurious pustules in cow were those similar to cowpox, but they belonged to another type of disease (a type of chicken-pox). They could give rise, if their lymph was inoculated in humans, to a "primary spurious vaccine" that was benign or malignant according to its virulence. This disease did not have any protective effect against smallpox (Sacco, 1809, pp. 72–5). Humans could have a spurious vaccine if the lymph used for vaccination was extracted from a degenerated (ulcerated) human vaccine pustule or from a bad site of a good pustule (in the centre, not in the border), which would elicit a "secondary spurious vaccine" (Sacco, 1809, pp. 76–85).

Addressing "the eyes" of his readers (Sacco, 1809, p. 10), Sacco published in his *Treatise* four coloured plates showing pustules in cow, horse, and sheep and real and spurious human vaccine (see Figs. 7–10). The plate of the pustules in the cow nipples was essentially the same as that his *Observation* (1801), in which the spontaneous and inoculation-induced pustules were represented (see Fig. 7). The plate about the horse sought to enable readers to distinguish grease from other similar eruptions in horses' hoofs, such as the "Crepazze", "Vesciconi", and "Ricciuoli" (Sacco, 1809, pp. 135–6). The real grease useful for vaccination was only the portion that affected the lateral part of the "pastern"; the lymph had to be extracted only at the beginning of the suppuration of the eruptions (Sacco, 1809, pp. 139–40). The plate showed the evolution of grease in three successive legs, with the preferred time point for extracting lymph corresponding to the central picture (Fig. 8).

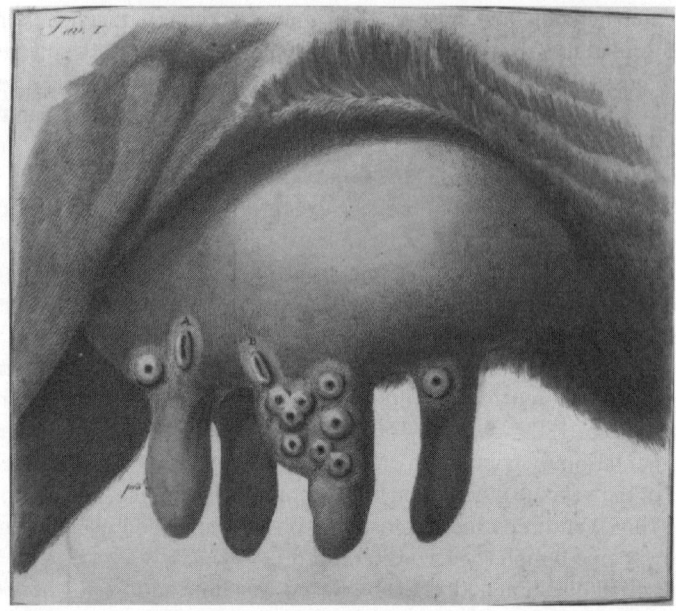

Fig. 7: vaccine pustules in cow with, down on the lefts, the detail of a pustule's profile ("pro")

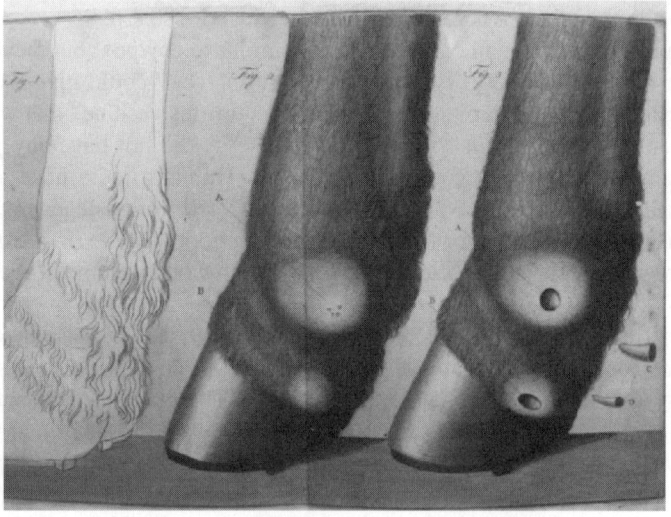

Fig. 8: evolution of pustules of "grease" in horse's leg

Sheep-pox was a disease in sheep similar to "Rogna" (scabies) or "Stizza" (Sacco, 1809, p. 148). Sheep-pox particularly affected the snout, and the pustules often formed groups (Sacco, 1809, p. 149). The corresponding plate for sheep clearly characterized the specific disease (Fig. 9).

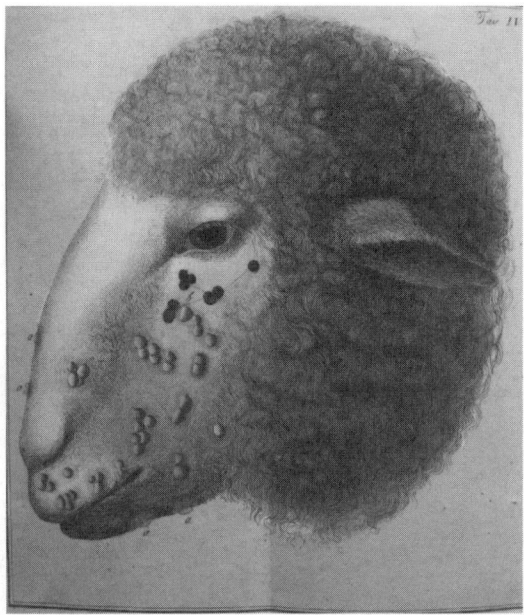

Fig. 9: pustules of sheep-pox with details of their profiles (on the left)

Finally, the plate for humans was probably the most detailed picture of real and spurious pustules available at that time. The plate showed two arms. The top arm showed the evolution of real vaccine from the beginning until the cicatrisation of the pustule. The bottom arm represented two different series of pustules, which showed the evolution of a "spurious malignant vaccine" or a "spurious benignant vaccine" (Fig. 10). The real vaccine pustules were more regular and less virulent than the spurious ones.

The four plates contained a new element compared to previous representations by Jenner and colleagues. Sacco showed not only the two-dimensional structure of the pustules and their evolution by a series of successive images, but also represented the profile of the pustules in cow, sheep, horse, and human. For example, in the image of the cow's udder, the first nipple from the left presented a small picture annotated with the word "pro" (for "profile"). The same inscription was found for the sheep (two small pictures on the left, under the noise, signed with two "a") and for human (12 small pictures on the border of the arms signed with "pr").

Just as the classical images of Jenner, Woodville, and Kirtland visualised the variables space and time, Sacco further developed the variable space. Sacco tried to represent in detail the three-dimensional structure of the pustules together with their profiles, an attempt which was a prelude to the full three-dimensional representation by wax models. The aim of this representation was even more specific than its predecessors: the image captured the specificity of the real vaccine pustule compared to the spurious one and also described where to extract the effective lymph

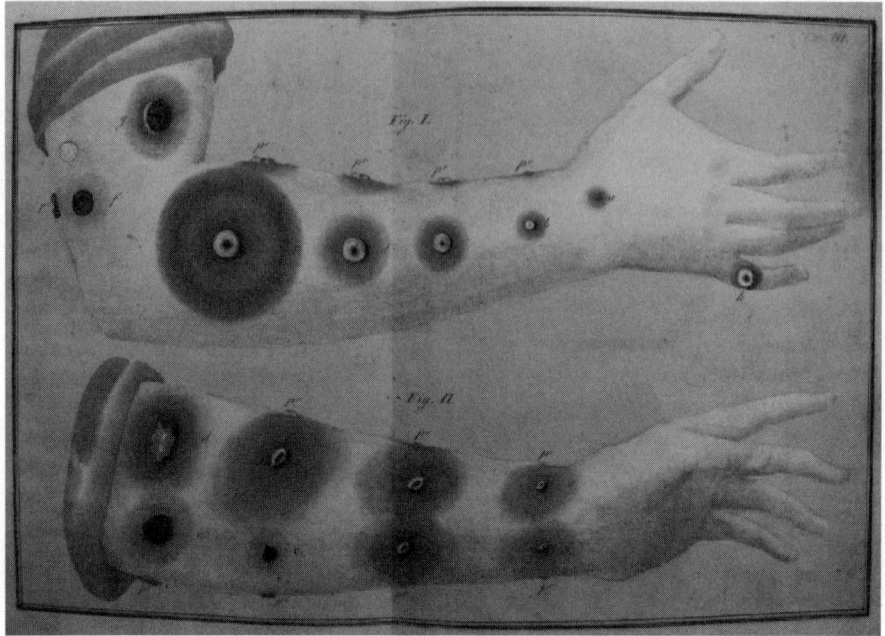

*Fig. 10: evolution of pustules of real (up) and spurious vaccine (down)
with details of their profiles*

for successful vaccination. The profile of the pustule showed a central depressed part covered with an eschar, while the border parts were more prominent and full of lymph. The careful vaccinator would take the good lymph from the border of the pustule. This knowledge could be fully transmitted only with a mixture of verbal descriptions and images, and Sacco deeply developed both of these aspects.

Our researches led us to find, in some north Italian hospitals and medical museums, a series of anatomical waxes that correspond exactly to the images from Sacco's *Treatise*. We have found the wax models in the archive of the Ospedale Maggiore in Milan, where Sacco started his medical carrier; in Cattaneo's Museum of Anatomical Waxes in Bologna (Aldini et al., 2007); in the Museum for the History of the University and the Museum of Pathological Anatomy in Pavia (Aldini et al., 2007, pp. 203–4); and in the Museum of Pathological Anatomy in Padua. The cities of Milan, Pavia, Bologna, and Padua belonged to the three different North Italy governments (Cisalpine Republic, Italian Republic and Italian Kingdom) in which Sacco was chief of vaccination. The waxes from these four cities are similar, and each is equipped with the same handmade explanation certifying that the models were produced under the direction of Pietro Moscati, a medical and political man related to Sacco.

The archive of the Ospedale Maggiore of Milan contains no trace of the origin of these wax models. The State Archive of Milan, in which is conserved the University Archive, is missing because of damage suffered by the building during the

Second World War. We can only attest to the presence of two wax models in the Ospedale Maggiore: one corresponding to Sacco's plate about cowpox, and one corresponding to the table about grease on horse.

Cattaneo's Museum of Bologna has two models, one representing cowpox in the nipples of cow and one representing two human arms that perfectly correspond to Sacco's plate. These two models are mentioned in the catalogue of the old Museum of Pathological Anatomy, which was written around the 1860s (Aldini et al., 2007, p. 197). The catalogue mentions, in total, four wax models representing cowpox, grease, sheep-pox, and human vaccine pustules exactly like those in Sacco's plates. It is reported that these models were donated to the museum by the Counsellor Moscati. Only two of these preparations have survived until today.

In Pavia, we found two models (cowpox and grease) in the Museum for the History of the University and a model of human arms in the Museum of Pathological Anatomy. In the State Archive of Pavia, there is a prospectus that describes these three models. The fourth model (of sheep-pox) is not mentioned here (Aldini et al., 2007, 203–4).

In the Museum of Pathological Anatomy of Padua, we found the complete series of four models (Figs. 11–14). There is full correspondence between Figs. 7 and 11, Figs. 8 and 12, Figs. 9 and 13, and Figs. 10 and 14. Each model is equipped with a handmade legend. Cowpox, grease, and human arms share the first common part of the legend: "Explanation of the vaccinal preparation contained in the three tables executed under the direction of Mr. Pietro Moscati, State Counsellor Consultant, Dignitary of the Order of Iron Crown, General Director of the Public Education."

Pietro Moscati graduated with a degree in medicine from the University of Pavia in 1758. In 1763, he obtained the chair of anatomy, surgery, and obstetrics at

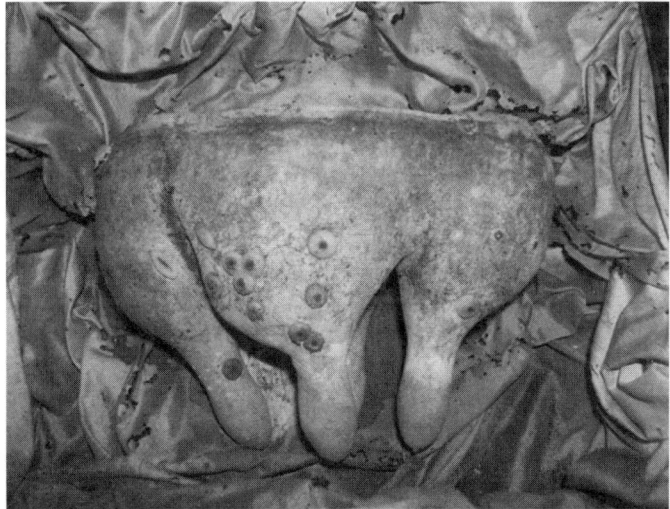

Fig. 11: wax model in the Paduan Museum of Pathological Anatomy
corresponding to the Plate I

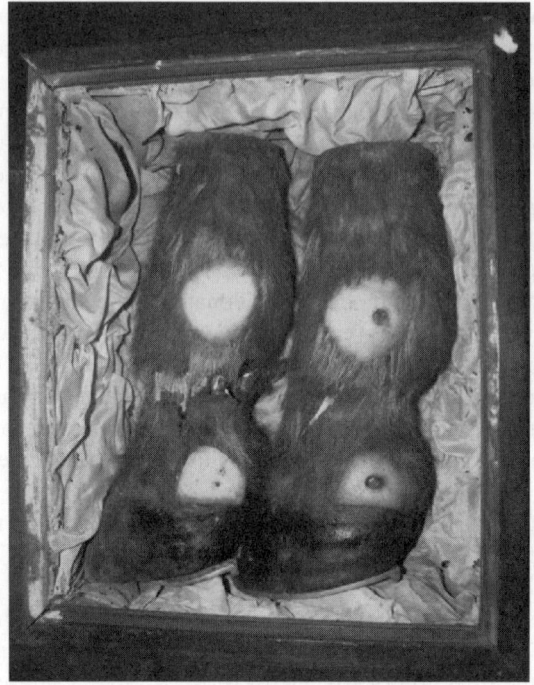

*Fig. 12: wax model in the Paduan Museum of Pathological Anatomy
corresponding to the Plate II of Sacco's Treatise (fig. 8)*

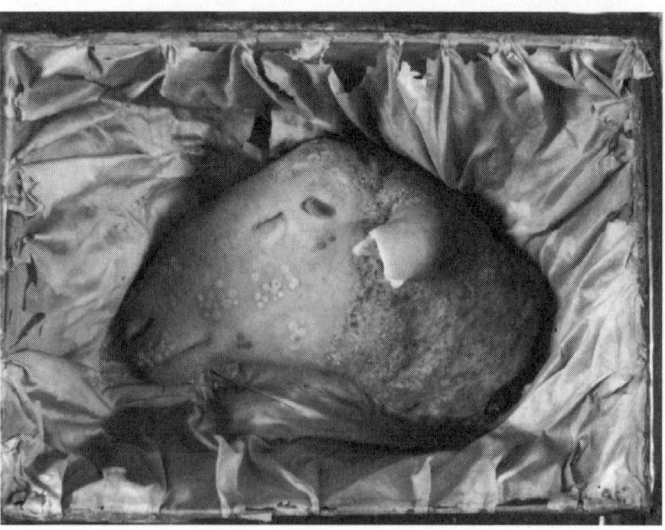

*Fig. 13: wax model in the Paduan Museum of Pathological Anatomy
corresponding to the Plate III of Sacco's Treatise (fig. 9)*

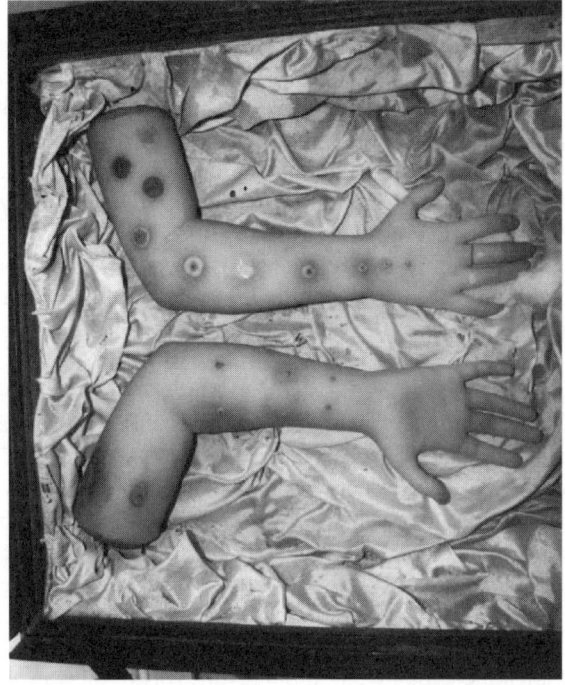

*Fig. 14 wax model in the Paduan Museum of Pathological Anatomy
corresponding to the Plate IV of Sacco's Treatise (fig. 10)*

the same University. In 1772, he became a professor of medicine and surgery at Milan Maggiore Hospital and director of the hospital in 1785. In 1796, he became member of the executive director of the "first" Cisalpine Republic (1797–1798). When Napoleon returned in 1800, Moscati became one of the major figures of political life during the "second" Cisalpine Republic (1800–1802), Italian Republic (1802–1805), and the Kingdom of Italy (1805–1814), and was named State Counsellor, Senator of the Kingdom, General Director of Public Education, and President of the Magistrate of Health (from 1805 to 1810) (Cosmacini, 1982, pp. 60–1). The Order of Iron Crown was an order of knighthood created by Napoleon in Milan in 1805, and Moscati was elected a dignitary in 1806.

Moscati showed an early interest in the didactic and scientific possibilities provided by wax modelling. This fact is testified in one of his books, in which he described the best ways for "preparing and conserving animal parts" (Moscati, 1785): "Between anatomical devices we have to list those of figuring with wax models the dissected parts of animal and the entire forms of muscles with so elegance and clearness that nothing is comparing" (p. 327). In 1781, the Austrian government, which at that time dominated North Italy, sent two apprentices to Florence to learn ceroplastic techniques. The aim was to return to Pavia and to create a collection of wax models "under the direction of professor Moscati" (Aldini et al., 2007, p. 203).

It is easy to understand why Moscati created the wax models of vaccination on the basis of Sacco's plates: he was a ceroplastic estimator and was the general director of public education and president of the magistrate of health from 1805 to 1810, the period in which Sacco was active and published his books. Moscati was interested in vaccination, as indicated by the fact that he was the first to practise the previous method of "variolation" in Milan (Belloni, 1962, p. 961). He also probably wrote an anonymous review of the Latin translation of Jenner's *Inquiry* published in Vienna in 1799 (Belloni, 1962).

What remains unclear is the relationship between Moscati and Sacco and whether we can consider Sacco to be a direct inspirer of this project. Sacco started his medical career at the Ospedale Maggiore of Milan, where he became Moscati's "friend" and "scholar" (Ferrario, 1858, p. 23; Ferrario, 1858a, p. 3). Moscati practised the first official variolation at a charity hospital in Milan ("Ospizio"), Santa Caterina della Ruota, in 1761. Sacco, at the same place in 1801, practised the first official vaccination: this act was a sort of "passing down of the title" between Moscati and Sacco. Finally, when Sacco was named general director of vaccination in 1801 by the Cisalpine Republic, Moscati was executive director of the government. This fact may imply that the presence of Moscati was essential in the nomination of Sacco. Given this strict relationship between Moscati and Sacco, we can safely postulate, even without the contribution of direct documentation, that Sacco inspired the creation of wax models. Furthermore, as noted above, Sacco recommended the establishment of "well-coloured drawings" or wax models in 1803 (Sacco, 1803, p. 36).

The legends of the ceroplastic preparations of cowpox found in Milan, Pavia, Bologna, and Padua all read as follows: "Nipples of cow with pustules of real vaccine and three other pustules of spurious vaccine." The legend of the wax models of the grease read: "Two horse's hoofs; one shows constitutional grease in the right time for giving the reproduction of vaccine. The other shows the same grease passed to suppuration and which doesn't be no more useful for the reproduction of vaccine." The legends of the wax models of the human vaccine pustules read: "The supine girl's arm represents two qualities of vaccine spurious; *benign* which terminates in six or seven days, and *malign* which produces a sort of anthrax. The arm in pronation present the *real vaccine* inoculated in winter which persists twenty-two days. It is signed by n. 11 graduate expulsions which shows their course each two days."

These legends correspond exactly to the explanations found in Sacco's *Treatise* of 1809. Regarding grease, for instance, Sacco wrote that the effective lymph for vaccination was to be extracted only at the beginning of the suppuration of the pustules and, in the explanation of the table, he defined it as "Constitutional grease in the period of suppuration" (Sacco, 1809, 224). Similarly, the legend of the wax model reports that the first horse's hoof represented the "constitutional grease in the right time for the reproduction of the vaccine". Regarding human vaccine, both wax models and Sacco's plate show three series of pustules: spurious malign, spurious benign, and real vaccine. Both the wax model's legend and Sacco's *Treatise* defined the spurious malign vaccine as a sort of "anthrax" (Sacco, 1809, p. 74).

Regarding the legend of the cowpox wax models and the cowpox plate in the *Treatise*, there is one significant difference. Both Sacco's plate and wax model represent two different types of pustules: one round and regular pustule, which is in the second frontal nipple from the left and is jointed in a system of three pustules; and one oval and extended pustule, which affects the first and second frontal nipples on the top (see Figs. 7 and 11). The legend of the wax models reports the representation of "three other pustules of spurious vaccine". Considering that "three pustules" are mentioned, one intuitively would think that these pustules are those shown as joined together in the second front nipple. In contrast, Sacco did not mention any spurious vaccine in his plate. Rather, he described the representation of the spontaneous pustules (the round and regular kind) and the two pustules that emerge from the inoculation of human vaccine lymph (the oval and extended ones) (Sacco, 1809, p. 222). These last pustules are indicated in the explanation of the plate with the letter "A".

Even more strangely, there is another inconsistency between the explanation given by Sacco on page 222 and his plate reproduced at the end of the book. In the explanation, he mentions two pustules by inoculation with the letter "A", while in the plate these two pustules are indicated with the letter "A" (the first on the left) and the letter "B" (on the right) (Fig. 8).

We have not been able to find a convincing interpretation of these inconsistencies between the wax model's legend and Sacco's plate and between Sacco's plate and Sacco's explanation. It is possible that Sacco forgot to explain pustule "B," which he eventually intended to have represent the spurious vaccine; however, this explanation is a very strange oversight for such a rigorous scientist. The author of the wax model's legend perhaps misunderstood this inconsistency and wrongly indicated the three round pustules as the spurious pustules. In any case, the lack of documented instructions for the creation of the wax models leaves us without any credible explanation. The perfect visual and structural correspondence between the plates and wax models remains.

In the Old Archive of the University of Padua, we found a document that states the precise date on which the wax models arrived in Padua from Milan. Only three models were produced under the direction of Pietro Moscati; the fourth wax model, representing sheep-pox and found in the catalogue of Bologna and at the Museum of Padua, had another history. The document consists of two letters sent by the prefect of the Department of "Brenta" – this department was the general administration of the Region of Padua – to the Regent of Padua University. The first document is a letter of presentation in which the prefect communicates to the regent of the university that he had received a "case", on 28 October 1807, from the "General Direction of the Public Education" of Milan, directed to the University of Padua (see Fig. 15).

The second letter is the verbal process redacted in the presence of Floriano Caldani (1772–1836), professor of anatomy of the University of Padua, and Marcantonio Galvani, chancellor of the same university. The letter reports as follows (Fig. 16):

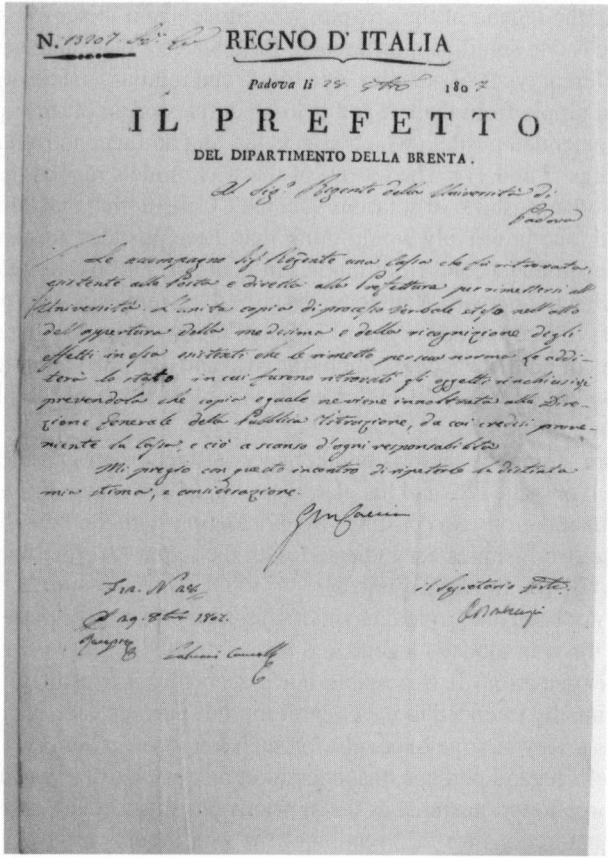

Fig. 15: letter of the Prefect of the "Brenta" attesting the reception of a "case"
from Milan for the University of Padua

[…] observed that [the case] was directed to the Mr. Prefect for sending it to the University, Mr. Professor of Anatomy Dr. Floriano Caldani and Marcantonio Galvani Chancellor of the University were invited, supposing that it was matter of anatomical objects. In the presence of these mysteries and opened the case, were find three cases containing explanations of vaccine preparations; the first, representing nipples of cow with pustules, having the crystal broken, for the rupture we saw introduced straws and dusts. The second, containing horse hoofs, not only presented the crystal broken in several pieces, but also we saw the preparations damaged at the point of being unusable. The third table, containing two girl's arms with pustules, had the hand's fingers detached and wandering in the case. […]

The descriptions clearly correspond to the models still conserved in the Padua Museum of Pathological Anatomy. The wax model of grease shows the first horse's hoof almost broken in two pieces, while the second hoof is quite damaged (see Fig. 12). The wax model of human vaccine pustules presents the first arm in pronation with two broken fingers: the middle and the ring fingers (see Fig. 14). What is

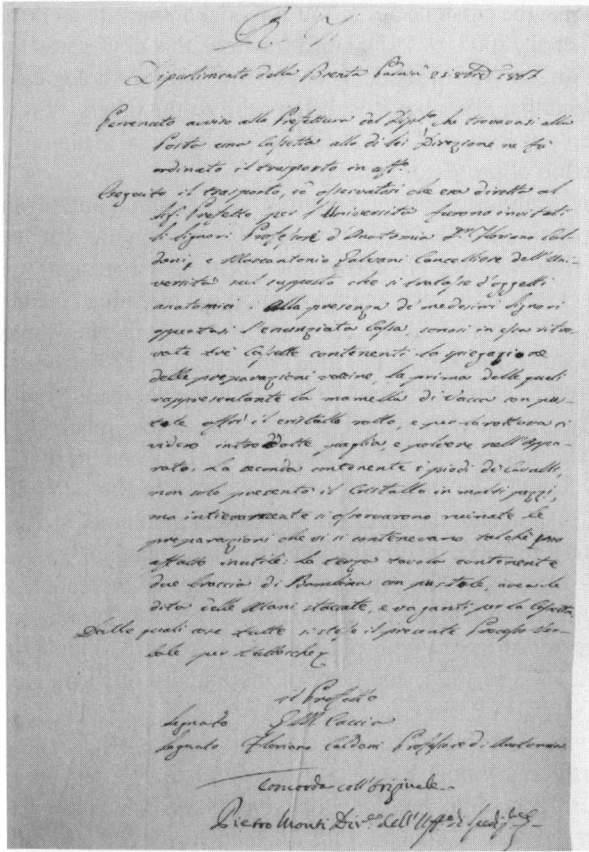

Fig. 16: report of the opening the case, revealing three wax models about vaccination

more interesting is the date of the document: 28 October 1807 corresponds to the period *after* the publication of *Memory* (1803), in which Sacco declared that the creation of plates and wax models was necessary, and *before* the publication of *Treatise* (1809), in which Sacco published his "well-coloured" plates. The wax models appear to have been a priority in the divulgation of Sacco's book, because they were created and distributed before them. The preparations were repaired and carefully conserved by the University of Padua, even if they were judged, at least the model of grease, as to be "unusable". This fact proves that they were used for their purpose, and that Caldani and Galvani were receptive about the purpose of these iconographical representations.

There is one more wax model that is not mentioned in the document of the Old Archive of the University of Padua or in the first part of the legend that is common for the first three models of Moscati. This fourth model is named in the catalogue of the old Bologna Museum of Pathological Anatomy, which reports, besides the other three preparations, the existence of a fourth model about "sheep-pox in a head of a sheep" (Aldini et al., 2007, p. 197). Unfortunately, this object was lost in Bologna, but in Padua a similar type of model is conserved in the Pathological Anatomy Museum. The legend that describes it is different from the others: "Preparation which shows the sheep-pox executed by Mr. Sandri – anatomical sculptor – the year 1819 under the direction of professor Fanzago."

We know almost nothing about this "Mr. Sandri", apart from the fact that he was a ceroplastic modeller from Bologna assumed by the University of Padua around 1816. However, we do know who "professor Fanzago" was. Francesco Luigi Fanzago (1764–1836) was an important figure of Paduan medicine in the first decades of the 19th Century. After obtaining a degree in philosophy at Padua in 1785, Fanzago studied medicine in Pavia from 1786 to 1789 (the same university where Sacco studied from 1786 to 1791) and in Padua again from 1789 to 1790, where he finally graduated in medicine. After the success related to his studies on pellagra and vaccination, in 1801, Fanzago was named as the "Protomedico dell'Ufficio di Sanità", an important position in the health administration of the town. In 1802, he obtained the chair of "theoretical medicine" at Padua University (Bertolaso, 1961). In 1806, he obtained the two first chairs in "pathology" and "legal medicine," instituted at the place of the old chair of theoretical medicine by a decree of the Director of Public Instruction Pietro Moscati (Bertolaso, 1961, p. 236). He was the director of the civil hospital of Padua from 1823 to 1830, rector of the university from 1823 to 1824, and dean of the Faculty of Medicine from 1828 to 1835.

We have not found any document attesting reasons why Fanzago decided to create the fourth wax model based on Sacco's plate. We presume that Fanzago knew Sacco during the time that they both studied medicine in Pavia. We also presume that Fanzago was in contact with Moscati for the creation of the chairs of pathology and legal medicine. Fanzago clearly was interested in the practice of vaccination, because he wrote a monograph on the topic in 1801 (Fanzago, 1801). It is known that he read and possessed Sacco's *Treatise*, because an original copy of this book belonged to his fund, which is now conserved in the Library "Pinali Antica" of the Faculty of Medicine. Fanzago was active in the creation and conservation of anatomical and anatomo-pathological specimens; he founded the first "Gabinetto Patologico" (pathological cabinet) around 1808 (Spongia, 1838, pp. 186–193). This cabinet became the Museum of Pathological Anatomy, in which his wax model is still conserved. We cannot analyse here the activity of Fanzago in vaccination and vaccination in Padua, which was important and was supported by the Austrian and French governments.

In 1819, twelve years after the reception of the wax models from Milan (in 1807) and 10 years after the publication of Sacco's *Treatise* (1809), Fanzago still felt the need to complete the series of waxes on vaccination by creating the model of sheep-pox (although we do not know whether the analogous fourth lost model of Bologna was inspired by Fanzago). We do not know whether these models were used directly by physicians and surgeons to study and practise vaccination, but the fact that Fanzago decided to create this waxwork proves that he approved the Sacco's project and that he was deeply receptive of the scientific and didactic importance of these tools.

LUIGI SACCO'S MEDICAL EPISTEMOLOGY

Luigi Sacco embodied the rising dimension of medicine that was imposed during the course of the 19th century. Sacco was not only a physician, but also a surgeon, and he expressed the typical "philosophy" of surgery: rejection of theoretical systems, absolute confidence in empirical observations, facts and experimentations, predilection for efficacy, and immediacy and practicality of therapeutic interventions, even without a complete theoretical demonstration. He wrote at the beginning of his *Treatise*:

> It has always been my opinion that the best way to reach esteem and reconnaissance from the public was to address his activity and research to the real advantage of the society, respecting those great men which dedicated in abstract and speculative studies [...]. It seems to me, however, that the first intention is better than the second when a good occasion arrives (Sacco, 1809, p. 5).

In this passage, Sacco shows his predilection for "action" and "research" against "speculative studies". The passage also shows Sacco's illuminist spirit, in his mention of the benefit of the humankind, "the real advantage of the society", judged to be better than any other type of speculation without a direct impact on the society.

Vaccination was a perfect domain for the expression of this epistemology. It was a simple and immediate practice that was empirically proven to be effective, also if it was not yet disposable the immunological knowledge for understanding its biological mechanisms. Vaccination was a testing ground for the new "democratic" ideal of health care. Sacco declared that "physicians, surgeons, and midwifes" could vaccinate. This statement enlarged the right to deal with an internal disease (i. e., smallpox) to surgeons, who normally were limited to the cure of external diseases, and to midwives.

Vaccination was also an ideal ground to battle against the old-style "systematic medicine". Several physicians belonging to this approach of medicine produced long series of theoretical objections against vaccination. One of the most important arguments was that smallpox was a spontaneous, internal disease by which the body purges itself of pathological humours. Sacco, in his *Treatise*, analyzed all of the objections to vaccination and proved their inconsistency from an empirical and experimental perspective (Sacco, 1809, pp. 191–211).

Regarding the lack of knowledge of the biological mechanisms of vaccination, Sacco explicitly elaborated his "epistemology of action": "We have to apply in the empirical research of the agents capable of producing natural phenomena, not to waste our time and to exhaust our mind in the research of the causes" (Sacco, 1809, p. 23). Throughout his book, Sacco repeatedly stressed: "If the simple philosopher is interested in the research of prime causes, practical physician remains satisfied when a series of several and constant experiences can give a sure and not misleading cognition of effects (even *a posteriori*)" (Sacco, 1809, p. 132). However, this position did not mean that he gave complete support to empirically based medicine bereft of any theory. On the contrary, Sacco repeated that his method was based on observations and experimentations, thanks to which he was able to deduce "some experimental truths" (Sacco, 1809, pp. 8–9).

The creation of the wax models was surely in line with this type of epistemology. Wax models were three-dimensional tools that fully expressed the ideals of immediacy and practicality that were constantly present in Sacco's books. The specificity of the knowledge of the vaccine was related to the observable structure of the pustules:

> The real vaccine lymph is in the interior of the pustule's cells, almost such as honey's in the honeycomb; and the spurious is in the cavity which constitutes the navel of the pustule, like in a separate follicle, prolonged in a way similar to a funnel and covered by an eschar (Sacco, 1809, p. 81).

Sacco recommended the development of "well-coloured drawings" and wax models, because it was "of the maximal importance" to be able to recognize real vs. spurious vaccine "even at the first sight" (Sacco, 1801, p. 194). His texts are disseminated with propositions related to the predominance of the visual aspect of knowledge, such as the importance "to acquire an eye" for recognizing the correct features of the pustules (Sacco, 1803, p. 36). The expression "to acquire an eye", literally translated from the Italian, corresponds to the English phrase "to get used".

Sacco's intention was to communicate not only with thinkers, but also and particularly with observers. Indeed, he declared that he prepared the "well-coloured drawings" on different pustules related to smallpox and vaccination in order to "speak better to the eyes of his readers" (Sacco, 1809, p. 10). To stress the importance of observation, he wrote that: "The inoculation of vaccine proves more than every other discovery how much experience and observation are necessary to sustain more evident the truths, and how feeble is in comparison the work of reasoning" (Sacco, 1809, p. 71). His purpose was to *show* the specificity of pustules in cow, horse, sheep, and human, to permit everybody to recognize them (Sacco, 1803, 36). Knowledge of this specificity was passed via the representation of the structure, colour, and time evolution of the pustules. At that time of history, without photography or television, there was nothing better than representation by ceroplastics, a technique already widely used for teaching anatomy and pathology.

Further research could reveal additional elements connected with the diffusion of these waxes in other Italian and European universities. The relationships between Sacco, Moscati, and Fanzago could be clarified with deeper research of the archives. Another interesting field to be explored is the eventual presence of images about vaccination in the medical and popular press and the presence of similar waxes in medical museums and expositions in the 19th century. We believe that this field could give some further insights into the diffusion and popularization of medical knowledge, a fundamental process to understand the constitution of the scientific credibility of medical sciences.

REFERENCES

AAVV, '*La ceroplastica nella scienza e nell'arte*', Atti del I Congresso Internazionale, Firenze 3–7 giugno 1975, 2 vols., Leo S. Olschki, Firenze.

Aldini, N.N., Pontoni, L., Scarani, P. and A. Ruggeri (2007), '*Documenti e immagini sull'innesto del vaiolo vaccino in Bologna al principio del XIX secolo*', *Medicina nei Secoli*, 19, 1: 195–208.

Anonymous (1800), '*A Comparative Statement of Facts and Observations relative to the Cow Pox published by Doctors Jenner and Woodville*', Sampson Law, London.

Belloni, L. (1962), '*La medicina a Milano dal Settecento al 1915*', in AAVV (1953–1966), *Storia di Milano*, Fondazione Treccani degli Alfieri per la Storia di Milano, Milano, vol. XVI: 933–1029.

Bertolaso, B. (1961), '*Francesco Luigi Fanzago (1764–1836) patologo e medico-legale nell'Ateneo padovano*', *Rivista di storia della medicina*, V, 2: 225–243.

Biagini, L. (1808), '*Rapporto storico-medico delle inoculazioni Ienneriane eseguite in Pistoja*', Stamperia Reale, Firenze.

Cosmacini, G. (1982) (ed.), '*Scienza medica e giacobinismo in Italia. L'impresa politico-culturale di Giovanni Rasori (1796–1799)*', Franco Angeli, Milano.

Fanzago, F.L. (1801), '*Memoria storica e ragionata sopra l'innesto del vajuolo vaccino*', Padova.

Ferrario, G. (1858), '*Vita ed opere del grande vaccinatore italiano dottore Luigi Sacco e sunto storico dello innesto del vajuolo umano del vaccino e della rivaccinazione*', Libreria di Francesco Sanvito, Milano.

Jenner, E. (1798), '*An Inquiry into the Causes and Effects of the Variolae Vaccinae: A Disease Discovered in some of the Western Countries of England, particularly Gloucestershire, and Known by the Name of the Cow Pox*', Sampson Low, London.

Jenner, E. (1799), '*Further Observations on the Variolae Vaccinae, or Cow Pox*', Sampson Law, London.

Jenner, E. (1800), '*A Continuation of Facts and Observations relative to the Variolae Vaccinae, or Cow Pox*', Sampson Law, London.

Jenner, E. (1800a), '*An Inquiry into the Causes and Effects of the Variolae Vaccinae: A Disease Discovered in some of the Western Countries of England, particularly Gloucestershire, and Known by the Name of the Cow Pox*', 2nd ed., Sampson Law, London.

Kirtland, G. (1802), '*30 Plates of the Smallpox and Cow Pox Drawn from Nature*', J. Jonson, London.

Maraldi, N.M., Mazzotti, G., Cocco, L. and F.A. Manzoli (2000), '*Anatomical Waxwork Modeling: The History of the Bologna Anatomy Museum*', *The Anatomical Record*, 261: 5–10.

McVail, J.C. (1896), '*Cow-Pox and Small-Pox: Jenner, Woodville, and Pearson*', *The British Medical Journal*, I: 1271–1276.

Morgagni, G.B. (1761), '*De sedibus et causis per anatomen indagatis libri quinque*', ex Thypographia Remondiniana, Venetiis.

Moscati, P. (1785), '*Appendice sui principali artifizj anatomici per preparare, e conservare le parti animali*', in Leske, G. (1785), *Elementi di storia naturale di N.G. Leske professore di storia naturale a Lipsia e membro di molte società scientifiche, ed economiche tradotti dal tedesco, aumentati, e migliorati da Ermenegildo Pini*, 2 vols, Imperial Monistero di S. Ambrogio Maggiore, Milano, vol. II: 305–332.

Pirson, C. (2009), '*For an Interdisciplinary Museology. The Particular Case of Anatomical Waxes*', *Medicina nei Secoli*, 21, 1: 91–115.

Sacco, L. (1801), '*Osservazione pratiche sull'uso del vajuolo vaccino, come preservativo del vajuolo umano*', Stamperia Italiana e Francese S. Zeno, Milano.

Sacco, L. (1803), '*Memoria sul vaccino unico mezzo per estirpare radicalmente il vajuolo umano diretta ai governi che amano la prosperità delle loro nazioni*', Stamperia e Fonderia De Stefanis, Milano.

Sacco, L. (1809), '*Trattato di vaccinazione con osservazioni sul Giavardo e vajuolo pecorino*', Tipografia Mussi, Milano.

Spongia, G. F. (1838), '*Di Francesco Fanzago nobile e medico padovano del suo secolo e de' suoi scritti*', Tip. Cartallier e Sicca, Padova.

Winkelstein W. (1992), '*Not just a Country Doctor: Edward Jenner. Scientis't*, Epidemiological Review*, 14, pp. 1–15.

MEDICAL IMAGING AND CONTEMPORARY ART: REDEFINITION OF THE HUMAN BODY

Katsiaryna Laryionava

> *'Freud and Jung made the inside of our heads fashionable. The inside of our bodies is still taboo.'[?]*
>
> Jeanette Winterson

INTRODUCTION

Röntgen's discovery of X-rays in 1895 made it possible to access the human body without dissection, thus dismantling its 'holiest' parts such as the sex organs and brain (Kevles 1997: 27); consequently, the idea was born that the human body can be completely transparent and visible for medical diagnoses without damaging its integrity (Van Dijck 2005). With this discovery, which according to Slatman initiated 'a new area', 'the Enlightenment of the body' (Slatman 2009: 107), it became possible to experience and to confront visually not only one's own inner body but also the bodies of others, producing a turning point from the use of anatomical images of dissected cadavers to the visualisation of the interior of the living body (Doyle 2007).

Since that time, many other more sophisticated computer-assisted medical imaging technologies such as computed tomography (CT), magnetic resonance imaging (MRI), positron emission tomography (PET), and ultrasound have been developed (Slatman 2009: 107) that are routinely used in current clinical practice. Furthermore, in today's media society, through the popularisation of medicine, these medical images have been disseminated into popular culture so that also the public can look inside the body, which was formerly the preserve of the medical profession. This has created what José van Dijck has called the 'myth of the transparent body' (Van Dijck 2005), i.e. the assumption that self-transparency means that the human body is more understandable or more familiar to everyone, and that these images can bring us closer to knowing what constitutes the human body.

By visualising the most intimate part of us, the interior of our body, these technologies have contributed to a new way of perceiving, experiencing, understanding, and defining our bodies (Slatman 2009: 107). Thus, they not only play an increasingly important role in clinical practice but also acquire a cultural presence and meaning, becoming a new influential phenomenon (Zwijnenberg 2010: 31; Van Dijck 2005: 9). This can be seen by the trend that many contemporary artists are becoming increasingly interested in the incorporation of medical images from their own or other's bodies into their work.

In the history of art, there has always been an exciting connection between the fields of art and science, in which art played an important role in the cultural dissemination of anatomical and physiological knowledge until the mid-19th century, when scientists and artists acted within the same intellectual sphere and shared the same philosophical and theological ideas (Zwijnenberg 2010: 31, 34). However, the present relationship and interactions between them has changed and the role of art goes far beyond the mere visualisation and dissemination of knowledge.

Notably, since the second half of the 20th century, artists have been increasingly working at the intersection of art and science, thus providing fertile ground for collaboration between these fields (Kemp and Wallace 2000: 6). This approach has helped to demolish the disciplinary barriers between, according to Snow, the once separated, even hostile to each other, 'two cultures' (Snow 1990), the (natural) sciences and the humanities. Although artists often, according to the media artist and theorist Jill Scott, utilise the same visualisation tools as scientists (Scott 2004), they do not interrelate with medicine in an illustrative way. Instead, blurring the borders between artistic and medical images, they explore, at the philosophical level, conceptual ideas within scientific medical discourse, creating new meanings and evoking ethical questions (Abbott 2006: 18).

The focus of this treatise is an artistic reflection of the human body through the use of medical imaging technology. Firstly, some artists' works that are based on new medical imaging technologies are discussed. Consequently, the following questions will be expounded: how does medical imaging change the perception, representation, and experience of the human body? How is the human body constructed and represented in art, and which bodies are thereby made visible for us? How has the representation of the body been changed by the development of more sophisticated medical imaging technology? What concepts of the human body do these artists transmit to us?

MEDICAL IMAGING TECHNOLOGIES AND ART

Since the second half of the 20th century, artists have been increasingly interested in using medical imaging to create self-portraits and to represent other people. These artists transform a medical image into an artistic pictorial representation and use their art to investigate the concept of the body, notions of self and identity, the relationship between what is virtual and what is real, the body and its image, and the vision and knowledge of the human body.

Early examples of artistic work that reflected on the representation of the body and the notion of identity which were created with the first medical imaging technology, the X-ray, include 'X-ray of Meret Oppenheim's Skull' (1964) by Meret Oppenheim, a Swiss surrealist artist, and Robert Rauschenberg's 'Booster' (1967), for which he X-rayed his entire body (Casini 2010). In these first attempts at using X-rays for artistic purposes, the human body appears to us as a constant image, and they were, therefore, similar to photography, i. e. directly mapping the human body. With the development of more sophisticated medical imaging techniques, such as 3-dimensional (D) and 4-D imaging, the representation of the body has profoundly changed.

Justine Cooper, an Australian-born new-media artist, works at the intersection of art, science, and medicine, bringing together animation, video, and installations with medical imaging technologies such as MRI to investigate the relationship between body, image, identity, and new medical technologies. In her computer video animation, RAPT I (1998), she used a series of MRI scans of her entire body in order to create an 'unmade and remade, dissected and reconstituted, in real time and in several orientations' (Cooper 2004: 188) self-portrait. The animation offers the viewer a trip into the artist's body, thus overcoming the borders of the physical body via technology (Gallasch 2003) and exploring the unknown sphere, i. e. the interior of the body, which, however, is not recognizable at first glance in the video. As the artist points out, 'The video, therefore, starts out inside my body, tracking through the interior of my leg until it breaches the boundary of inside and out when the 'camera' pulls out of the collarbone. At this stage the viewer becomes aware it is a body they are looking at. This body is then choreographed within its own space-time framework...melting, and then reconstituting itself...compressing and expanding, decaying and rebuilding' (Donohue 1999).

In a further work, entitled RAPT II (1998), she continued to experiment with MRI scans of her body, which had been scanned and reconstructed on a computer screen. Edited images of her body were printed onto 76 transparent sheets hanging sequentially in a room, thereby creating a 10-metre long 2-D data-body sculpture (Cooper 2004: 188). In this installation, Cooper transforms the 'living flesh' into 'malleable data' (Cooper 2004: 188), which can be reconstructed by the viewer moving around the installation. In this way the whole dismembered body can be reconstructed; however, the viewer must move around the figures in order to completely understand the full body image.

An English artist, Angela Palmer, in collaboration with scientists, used MRI scans to create a series of self-portraits. Processed on a computer, MRI scans of her body were hand-engraved on transparent non-reflective sheets of glass, which were placed one above the other, thereby building layers of lines and creating a translucent image. The portrait, as a whole, can only be perceived when the viewer stands in a particular location (Casine 2010). Furthermore, these 'self-portraits' could be construed as being anyone by the viewer.

Yet another British artist, Marilene Oliver, also used different medical imaging technologies, such as CT, MRI, and PET, of her own body and of anonymous subjects to create her artworks. In her 3-D sculpture, 'I Know You Inside Out' (2001), she 'rebuilt' the body of a man, Joseph Paul Jernigan, who was a convicted killer. She 'put him back together again', (Oliver 2007) by using pre-existing CT and MRI scans of his body, which were downloadable from the internet. She printed these images onto transparent acrylic pieces, which were then used to recreate his full body image, 'relocated in time and space, returned from a digital to an analogue state' (Oliver 2007).

In her 'Family Portrait' she made life-sized sculptures of her father, mother, sister, and herself, also based on MRI scans. These transparent sculptured portraits were generated with a similar technique as that used for the Jernigan piece. Oliver screen-printed the MRI images of her family members, which were layered on top

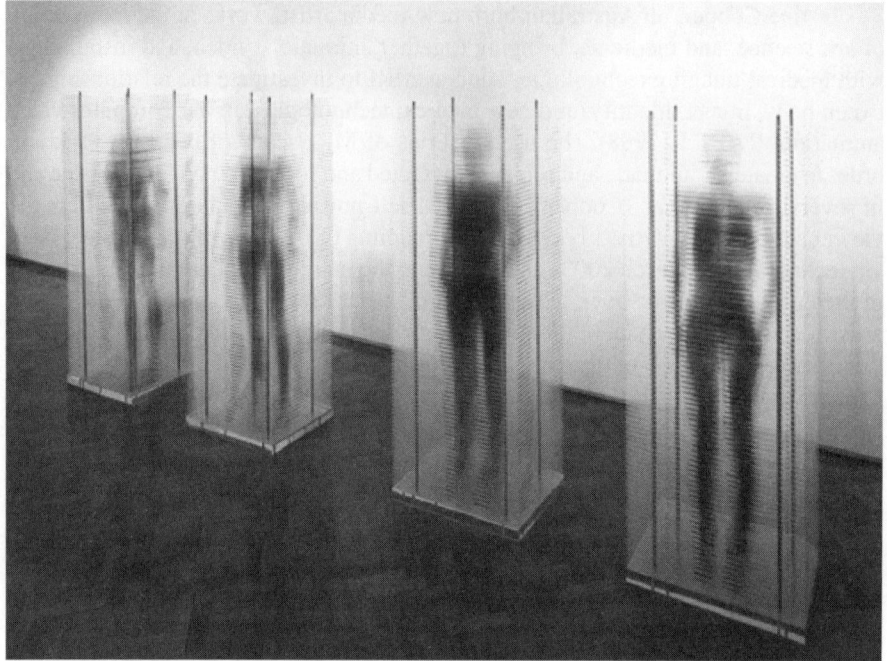

Fig. 1. Marilene Oliver Family Portrait (2003)

of each other on clear acrylic sheets, thereby reconstructing the scanned, fragmented body data. On the basis of the same principle used in the other works, the installation allowed the viewer to visualize the entirety of the transient body depending on their vantage point (Oliver 2007).

A further series of sculptures by Oliver, 'Dervishes', were made from CT scans, but not of the artist's own body. CT scans cannot be used for non-medical purposes, as the body is radiated during the scan; therefore, Oliver used a CT dataset of an anonymous female, whom she named MELANIX, which she downloaded from the internet. Thus, the physical body was transformed into a virtual one, which could be 'manipulated, sliced, rendered and surfaced' through artistic means (Oliver 2007).

Mona Hatoum, a Lebanese artist living in London and Paris, used endoscopic images of her own body in her video installation, 'Corps étranger' (Foreign Body) (1994). The installation consists of a white cylinder with 2 entrances. On the floor of the cylinder visitors see a circle with moving video images, which are hard to decipher at first. However, after having entered the cylinder, it becomes clear that the interior of the human body is being depicted, although only moving fragments of the body can be identified. The viewer experiences Hatoum's body through the lens of the medical camera. Simultaneously, the viewer can grasp that they are observing the image of a body, which could be the viewer's own body.

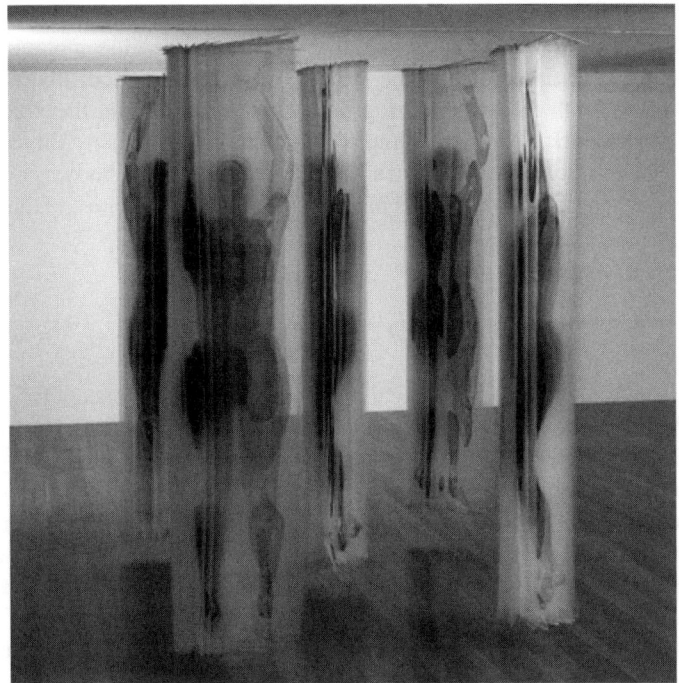

Fig. 2. Marilene Oliver Dervishes (2007)

ART AND THE CONCEPT OF THE HUMAN BODY

With the emergence of advanced medical imaging technologies, the representation and perception of the human body within the scientific community and cultural discourse has changed. Artists working with medical imaging technologies contribute to the reflection upon the visual experience of our interior, thereby helping us to approach an understanding of the role of technology in the conception of embodiment.

Although artists incorporate representations of their own or another's body in different ways, it becomes apparent upon viewing their artworks that there are common, identifiable formative motifs which reflect the concept of the body mediated through medical imaging technologies. Through this transition of the body from medical images into artistic representations, a definite concept of the body is conveyed to viewers.

THE FRAGMENTED BODY

In all these artworks, the body does not appear as an entire, constant image which can be precisely defined and easily recognized by the viewer. On the contrary, it appears either fragmented and consisting of different parts or scanned slices which are layered in order to create the impression of the whole body image or it is in a permanent state of flux, changing its form and position while metamorphosing, making the identification of its fragments possible, yet making it difficult to identify the whole body. Both the artist, during the artistic process, and the viewer, while observing the artwork, deconstruct and reconstruct the body many times over, and the body in its entirety is transient. In some of these works, the body as a whole can only be seen when the viewer stands in a specific place or watches it from a certain angle.

THE BODY AS A DATASET

In comparison to photography, medical imaging technologies, except for X-rays, do not reproduce the body image directly, but rather create a complex set of computed constructed data which require highly trained skills to be interpreted by medical professionals (Smelik 2010: 10; Schinzel 2006). Adopting this idea, artists use medical body images as portions of data that can be manipulated, combined, disassembled, reconstructed, copied, or otherwise edited. They re-define the portrait, which simultaneously becomes a visual representation of the body and a set of medical data. Artists do not focus on external physiological markers of the body that are used to construct our sense of self or identity, but rather penetrate the surface, as they are interested in converting the body to data and the data back to the body; thus, they change the body into a reconstructable, copied, informational, immaterial body. Furthermore, it involves the increased participation of viewers to interpret the created image, which is similar to the role of a medical professional, whose interpretation is necessary to understand the image.

THE 'ALIENATED' BODY

Artists investigate the perception of identity, and consequently indicate the ambiguity between what we perceive while looking at these body images and making a determination about them, and what we feel upon viewing them; thereby asking whether these body images are a means of identification or disidentification. The body images transmitted in the artworks appear to not be particularly familiar and easy to identify with, but rather estranged, alienated, and separated. In addition, these images appear intimidating and disturbing, make our bodies foreign to us, and expose the gap between the certainty of its physical presence and the uncertainty of its concept; as the German artist Timm Ulrichs stated, 'The deeper we look into ourselves, […], the more mysteriously, abysmally, eerily and strangely we appear to ourselves and we realize what we are: a foreign body' (Gockel 2008: 53).

CONCLUSION

The use of medical imaging technologies by artists demonstrates that the scanned inner body has become a complex, cultural construction which challenges our experience of the body and physicality, as well as our notion of self-identity and provokes questions on the cultural level such as how to integrate our body's interior image into our general notion of body and self (Zwijnenberg 2010: 31).

Medical imaging technologies have made our body transparent without damaging its integrity, thus creating a 'myth of the transparent body' (Van Dijck 2005). Artists challenge this notion in their works and the idea that seeing is equated with knowing and understanding. Exposing the lightness of its layers and borders, while fragmenting and virtualising each part, artists show that the body becomes transparent, but not necessarily more comprehensive.

Their artworks do not transmit a clearly defined idea of the human body that is easy to identify with. They are fragmented and transient with fluid boundaries between the body and the outside world, and appear indefinite and problematic, thus offering us increased uncertainty about our bodies and physicality.

REFERENCES

Abbott, Wynn (2006) 'Feature: Medical Interventions – Visual Art meets Medical Technology', The Lancet 368: 17–8.

Casini, Silvia (2010) 'The Aesthetics of Magnetic Resonance Imaging (MRI): from the Scientific Laboratory to an Artwork', Contemporary Aesthetics, Accessed on 20 May 2010, http://www.contempaesthetics.org/newvolume/pages/article.php?articleID=569#FN17.

Cooper, Justine (2004), 'Rapt', in, Tofts, D., Jonson, A. & Cavallaro, A (eds.) Prefiguring Cyberculture: An Intellectual History: 188–90.

Donohue, Robyn (1999) 'Photofile – Justine Cooper: RAPT', Accessed on 20 May 2010, http://www.justinecooper.com/donohue.html.

Doyle, Julie (2007) 'Cybersurgery and Surgical (Dis)embodiment: Technology, Science, Art and the Body', Transformations 15, Accessed on 20 May 2010, http://www.transformationsjournal.org/journal/issue_15/article_03.shtml.

Gallasch, Keith (2003) 'Justine Cooper: New Media Alchemist. Keith Gallasch emails Justine Cooper in New York', Real Time 55 (June – July), Accessed on 20 May 2010, http://www.realtimearts.net/article/55/7081.

Gockel, Cornelia (2008) 'Reise zum Ich Der Blick in das Innere des Körpers in der Kunst nach 1960', Innovation 19(3): 50–3.

Kemp, Martin & Wallace, Marina (2000) 'Spectacular Bodies. The Art and Science of the Human Body from Leonardo to Now' (Berkeley, Los Angeles, London).

Kevles, Holtzmann Bettyann (1997) 'Naked to the Bone: Medical Imaging in the Twentieth Century' (New Brunswick: Rutgers University Press).

Oliver, Marilene (2007), 'Resurrecting the Digitised Body: The use of the 'Scanned in' Body for making Artworks', EVA London 2007: 15.1–15.10. EVA Conferences International, Accessed on 26 November 2010, http://www.marileneoliver.com/writings/writpubpapers.html.

Scott, Jill (2004) 'Interview von Yvonne Volkart mit der Medien-Künstlerin und Theoretikerin Jill Scott über Fantasien von einem Erweiterten Körper als einem Morphologischen und Relationalen Körper'. Accessed on 12 May 2010, http://www.medienkunstnetz.de/themen/cyborg_bodies/erweiterte_koerper/.

Schinzel, Britte (2006) *'The Body in Medical Imaging between Reality and Construction'*, *Poiesis und Praxis* 4(3): 185–98. Accessed on 20 May 2010, http://mod.iig.uni-freiburg.de/cms/fileadmin/publikationen/online-publikationen/med.im.construct.pdf.

Slatman, Jenny (2009) *'Transparent Bodies: Revealing the Myth of Interiority'*, in Van De Vall, R. & Zwijnenberg, R. (eds), *The Body Within: Art, Medicine and Visualization* (Brill's Studies in Intellectual History) (Brill Academic Pub): 107–23.

Smelik, Anneke (2010) *'Introduction – The Scientific Imaginary in Visual Culture'*, in Smelik, A. (eds.) *The Scientific Imaginary in Visual Culture (Interfacing Science, Literature, and the Humanities)* (V&R Unipress): 9–21.

Snow, Charles Percy (1990), *'The Two Cultures'*, Leonardo, 23 (2/3) 169–173.

Van Dijck, Jose (2005) *'The Transparent Body: A Cultural Analysis of Medical Imaging'* (In Vivo: *The Cultural Mediations of Biomedical Science*) (University of Washington Press).

Winterson, Jeanette (2003) *Intimate Distances*, Accessed on 20 May 2010, http://www.marileneoliver.com/writings/writexhibessayswinterson.html.

Zwijnenberg, Robert (2010) *'How to Depict Life: A Short History of the Imagination of Human Interiority'*, in Smelik, A. (eds.) *The Scientific Imaginary in Visual Culture* (Interfacing Science, Literature, and the Humanities) (V&R Unipress): 21–39.

IMAGE – BODY – KNOWLEDGE: AN INTERDISCIPLINARY AND CRITICAL APPRAISAL OF IMAGES

Richard Hoppe-Sailer, Rainer-M. E. Jacobi, Sarah Sandfort

PREFACE

After various preliminary discussions, a workshop entitled "Image – Body – Knowledge" occurred in December of 2009, at the Kulturwissenschaftliches Institut (KWI) in Essen. The workshop was initiated in cooperation between the KWI, the Medizinhistorisches Institut of the Universität Bonn, the Kunsthistorisches Institut of the Ruhr-Universität Bochum, and the Medical Solutions sector of Siemens AG (Healthcare, Erlangen).[1] The parties involved met with representatives of various medical fields and discussed the tasks, objectives, and work structure of the planned project. The following article presents the results of the workshop associated with the project.

1. ABSTRACT

This project is focused on modern medical imaging techniques and images. The increase in knowledge and diagnostic or therapeutic competence provided by visual representations is crucial in the field of medicine. Medical images comprise an important part of the diagnosis and therapy process; the use of these images frequently makes the difference between health and disease or between life and death. The current state of research in different fields, such as visual culture, art history, philosophy, science, and media studies, shows the indetermination and the uncertain realism of the image. Central to these discussions are questions about the status and concept of the image: Is the image a sign (and, if so, what kind of sign), as semiotic theories propose? Or does the image have its own reality separate from its material basis, as phenomenological theories propose? Neither medicine nor visual culture studies nor *image sciences*[2] are sufficiently concerned with the "iconic paradigm" of their images.

The status and significance of computer-generated images is very important in terms of the generation of medical knowledge (such as in university teaching or

---

1 See the publication of the article '*Your Body: in the Focus*' (Peter Allegretti) in *Medical Solutions* (Siemens AG), May 2011: 62–67.

2 This term does not refer to the "image science" of W. J. T. Mitchel, but rather is an attempt to translate the German phrase "Bildwissenschaften". In this study, the term "image studies" refers to disciplines that are interested in questions about images.

research) and the physician-patient interaction. In medicine, computer-generated images represent a crucial media type whose social, political, and ethical implications are inconceivable in their scope. The thesis of this project is that a specific and critical appraisal of medical images is needed: namely, a critical appraisal related to particular modern medical imaging techniques (e. g., computed tomography [CT] and magnetic resonance imaging [MRI]) and to the anthropological notions of the medical application of the images.

The first step in the critical appraisal of an image is to clarify the different steps in the corresponding imaging techniques, and the changes that they invoke on the representation of the original object (i. e., the body). Since the development of computer-based imaging methods such as CT and, especially, MRI, the status of the generated images has been questioned. The continuum between the observed object, the act of observation, and the resulting image gets lost, because the results (i. e., the images) can no longer be compared directly with the object (i. e., the human body). In cases where the image is the result of in vivo techniques, a comparison with the object is impossible. In other cases, perfection of the imaging techniques prevents a comparison with the object, because the images are "better than reality" in their resolution and virtual realisation.

Computer-generated imaging techniques are associated with a loss of the epistemic and aesthetic continuum; this situation distinguishes modern medical imaging techniques from artistic images and classical scientific images (e. g., microscopy images). The latter are still seen as "images," whereas the generation process is hidden in the computer-generated outcomes. The technical development of images with such modern medical imaging techniques produces results that are not representative of reality; complex mathematical calculations and image processing are performed that are not obvious in the final product. Additionally new imaging techniques increase the possibilities of manipulation: traditional visual experiences and presumptions could enter the imaging process, change the results, and make the status of the image (e. g., as copy *of* or sign *for* the object) difficult to determine.

There is a peculiar absence of images of diseased humans and changes in the way of representation of the human body in modern medical imaging. In the context of images, this absence and changes intensify the occurrence of paradox. Positive – particularly false positive – findings could lead to a quasi "virtual construction" of the disease. The diseased human is no longer the cause, but rather the "result" of imaging.

The perfection of computer-generated images also affects our concept of the human body. Physicians work with concepts of normativity, so-called "standard images", which are often generated by software programs and with statistical methods. Until now, the ethical context has focused on a descriptive concept of disease rather than on a normative concept. The normative concept covers the dignity of the individual anamnesis, because the disease of one person is generalized in statistical procedures. This aspect is increased by modern imaging techniques. Medical diagnoses are increasingly being determined by normative ideas of disease: namely, through standard images. According to Habermas (Habermas 2001: 43–125), there is a difference between "technischer Herstellung" (technical manufacture) and "klinischer Einstellung" (clinical setting), which suggests the problem of using normativity or standardized images in medicine: Habermas means a methodical separation between (standardized) disease and individual life in modern medicine. Basing our understanding of disease and of the human body on technical innovations can lead to extensive ethical questions in medicine.

This project addresses 1) the interplay of several disciplines regarding their adaptability for diagnostic-therapeutic processes, and 2) the development and practice of an internal model for the critical appraisal of images. The tasks involved in this critical appraisal include determining the technical disembodiment (i. e., the lost relationship between the human body itself and the image representing it) and researching the influence of the verbal interpretation of digital images on the generation of medical knowledge.

The model of critical appraisal must deconstruct some inherent prejudices. Not only must the model assess how physicians and scientists speak about artefacts of new imaging techniques, it also must address how this speaking about artefacts (i. e., the medical images) creates again an *artefact* in linguistic interpretation. The term *artefact* is derived from art-historical terminology, and not medical terminology. When a physician refers to an artefact, he or she means the image distortions generated through the imaging techniques or errors in the setting. In contrast, for the art historian, the existence of an artefact means that the production of the image was influenced by a person involved in the imaging process and that the image is not a representation of reality but creates an own meaning. Similarly the linguistic interpretaion of images constructs another meaning or another reality than the image and seems an artefact itself.[3] Therefore apart from questions about the terminology of different fields the speaking about images is a part of the research on the critical appraisal of images.

Neither diagnostic findings nor therapeutic interventions are able to use images without verbalizing them. Images are also important in the physician-patient relationship, where both individuals must speak about the image. The difference between the physician (as a professional) and the patient (as a layman) is reflected in their speech about and their usage of images. Similarly, images structure the social fabric in hospitals and clinics; for example, who is allowed to produce/read/etc. the images? This social impact is reflected in speech as well.

The planned project connects the concrete physician-patient relationship with the discussion of iconographic matters and methods of image generation, and it also connects the speech of image description and anamnesis with critical deliberations of the epistemological status of medicine. The objective is to obtain a theoretically based and empirically validated determination of the importance of medical imaging. Implicit in this determination of importance are the consequences on health policy, financial economics, medical technology, and medical ethics.

---

3 The different "levels of reality" could depend on different media types. But the problem is the transfer between reality (i. e., the body in medicine), image (i. e., the diagnostic image), and language (i. e., the medical report) which is so far unreflected.

2. CURRENT STATE OF RESEARCH

The critical appraisal of medical images was arranged with respect to the relationship between the image, the object (i. e., the body), and knowledge. This critical appraisal is influenced by not only visual culture studies, but also by cultural history, anthropology, and social politics. The broad field, from technical imaging to its medical application, constitutes the specific problem of the project. Indeed, the project is focused on the history and current use of images, on data processing and aesthetics, on visualization and narration, on representativeness and physicality, as well as on perception and operation. At the same time, these various attributes reflect that the study is an indeterminate and implicit transdisciplinarity.

In a conventional interdisciplinarity, it is characteristic to ask for the methods; for the current project, it is characteristic to ask for the object. A critical appraisal of images has as its object not only the images themselves, but also the technical and cultural conditions of their genesis, the situation and history of the physician and patient, and the motifs, expectations, and procedures of the imaging process. Because the research of humans constitutes the humanization of medical-technical innovations – as described before in reference to the problem of normativity and the human treatment of individuals – this project also belongs in the field of cultural studies.

Radical changes that have occurred in the last 2 centuries influence any fundamental discussion of image, sight, and view. The idea of an "image" (among other things) is embedded in the context of digital technology. New approaches to the terms and theories of images (pictorial/iconic turn) and to the relationship between image and speech are needed (Boehm 1994; Mitchell 1994, 2008). Particularly in biology and medicine, the history of science is synonymous with the history of the image (Breidbach 2005; Foucault 1973). For the medical appraisal of images, anthropological approaches are combined with semiotic and phenomenological approaches of modern image science. Questions in such appraisals concern the image location, the practical use of images, and the implications provided by images. The anthropology of images becomes the paradigm of interdisciplinary cultural sciences (Belting 2001; Foucault 1971; Wiesing 2005).

In terms of digital image generation in the 20th and early 21st century, the media type and iconicity of technical images are important, as are e. g. the construction and visualization of the invisible (Breidbach 2000; Merleau-Ponty 1964) or the loss of the iconic and epistemological continuum between the object and viewer through experimental conditions of image generation (Adelmann/Frercks 2009). The digital visualization of invisible objects – like the interior body in medicine – often arises without causally determined connection between image and object. The references of images are more experimental data instead of the human body. So the notion "iconicity" becomes uncertain and depends on the limits and conditions of media types.

A review of the history of medicine reveals that there has been a radical change in the media (hand, ear, or eye) used to influence the modern medical appraisal of images. A critical appraisal of the image addresses the ontological and anthropological differences between the image and body, as well as between a specific moment and history. Questions about the reality of technical images (Baudrillard 2000) or about the technical and visual reduction of the body to a disembodied picture (Belting 2002, 2004) have extensive consequences for the interpretation and the epistemological status of (medical) images (Heintz/Huber 2001; Stahnisch/Bauer 2007).

The supposed objectivity of medical image generation can be part of the socio-cultural development of facts and knowledge (Daston/Galison 2007; Fleck 1983). The affirmative character and the suggestive factuality of technically optimized images can lead to a loss of knowledge through an increase of information: false-positive results, image models, and development of hypotheses (Breidbach 2006; Hagner 1996). The tension between the logic of images ("ikonische Episteme") and the binary decision-making structure of physicians is the basic problem of image-based diagnostic techniques (Boehm 2007, 199 ff.; Heßler/Mersch 2009).

With their attainment of technical and aesthetic perfection, medical images have lost their status as signs: theoretical models serve as references and not as empirical results (Breidbach 2006; Bredekamp/Werner 2003). A normative inversion of the world and the image results from this scenario (Heidegger 1980) and important terms like "normality" and "abnormality" have become elements of the image generation (Stahnisch/Bauer 2007). The medical results for the individual or the individual "normativity of the living"[4] (Canguilhem 1974; Weizsäcker 1997) can be interpreted as pathological through statistical constructed standards (or standard images). Consequently, the medical appraisal of images requires the contextualization through a concrete anamnesis (Jacobi 2008) to prevent a (false) pathologising of healthy individuals. The cultural history of the practice, effect, and power of human images is becoming more important from an ethical context (Burri 2008).

3. DESCRIPTION OF THE PROJECT

The starting point for this project was a prominent desideratum of previous research: namely, questions about the generation, status, and application of modern technical imaging methods in medicine. Our interest was focused on digital image processing techniques and CT or MRI image generation. People from various disciplines were involved in the December 2009 workshop, including researchers in art history, philosophy, industrial design, psychosomatics, neurology, neuroradiology, clinical anatomy, orthopaedics, and others. These individuals determined the structure and organization of the project as well as its questions.

The parties involved agreed that various assumptions and preliminary decisions are – often unconsciously from the actors – integrated into image generation, and that they cannot be reconstructed from the image itself. Therefore, the generation of

---

4   The "normativity of the living" means that every individual has an experience of disease which gets lost in the objectivated notions and practices about disease in modern medicine.

images is ethically and clinically questionable, because the parameters that can affect the outcome of the medical imaging often are not obvious. This situation is associated with the questionable iconic and ontological status of the images. The images have a fascinating realism that leads to a peculiar paradox: the increasing amount of information (by digitalization, resolution, and colouring) causes a loss of reference and reality. It becomes unclear whether the image actually functions as an image, in terms of semiotic theories, when a "visual reductionism" is in effect. The relationship between an image, the body, and knowledge is the central issue of this research.

The question of the source and place of normativity when dealing with computer-generated images is important for their clinical application. The visualization of otherwise invisible phenomena leads to the scenario in which models and other images, rather than the object (e. g., the human body), become sources for the concept of normativity. Positive and negative findings must be correlated with physical results in the context of individual anamneses. The unexplored relationship between normativity and pathogenicity is a fundamental deficit of previous research and practice in the clinical application of medical imaging. The iconic, disciplinary, and anthropological contexts are conditions for legitimate interpretations of medical images, but these contexts still are only insufficiently reflected.

We sought to provide an empirically validated contribution to the research of medical practice with images and to establish a self-reflective pictorial concept or concept of images. A critical appraisal of images requires a systematic analysis of the genesis, status, and application of medical imaging. This critical appraisal implies not only a new form of interdisciplinarity that varies from mathematical formalisms of imaging to psychosocial dynamics of images in the physician-patient communication, but also influences the cultural, socio-political, and ethical status of modern medicine. The objectives of the project are 1) the development of a medical understanding of images, and 2) the design of concepts for product responsibility on the part of the manufacturer of medical imaging systems.

4. PRESENTATION OF THE COLLABORATORS
(IN THE STRUCTURE OF THE PROJECT)

The development of a critical appraisal of images depended on the collaboration of the different cooperating partners. The relationship between image, body, and knowledge opens many questions within various disciplines. The involved parties in the workshop divided the research field into 3 main parts: image, body, and society. *Image* addressed questions pertaining to the media type of images (reference, iconicity, etc.) and to the history, technical manufacture, and design of the medical image. *Body* referred to the relationships between image and body and image and knowledge. The relationship between image and body affects the body-awareness, the concepts of *Self* and *Other*, the visualization of invisible phenomena etc. The relationship between image and knowledge involves aspects of normativity, epistemology, and ontology. *Society* also is concerned with relationships. The relation between image and speech is important for the communication between the physician and patient in terms of concept formation, diagnosis, and therapy. Similarly, the relationship between image and culture affects the history of seeing and the medical consciousness of images, similar to imagination and perception. Finally, the relationship between image and public influences the practical use of images, the competence of the critical appraisal, and justice and rights (e. g., health insurance).

All of the cooperating partners will research different areas in the study, and the results will be collected regularly. The Kunsthistorisches Institut in Bochum is interested in the medical image in its mediality, and it will research the relationship between the image and object: in particular, the problem of reference, the image's character as a sign, and its iconicity and temporality (defined as the comparison between the time of the object and time of the image). The status and concept of the (technical) image, the technical implications of image generation, and the process of medical imaging between mimesis, simulation, and construction are all of interest. The Institute researched the implications that the image's indetermination has on pictorial knowledge and assessed the relationship between the experience of the own body and the body's representation in virtual images.

For image analysis, the context of specific medical images is important. The Medizinhistorisches Institut of the Universität Bonn and the Anatomische Anstalt of the Universität München will address the history of medical imaging and research image traditions and influences of the actor's expectations of the images. Of interest are process-related differences between X-ray and nuclear spin, structural and functional imaging, or analogue and digital image generation. In both institutions, curricula for the medical competence of the images are planned as supplements to the study of history, theory, and ethics in medicine. Questions about the mediality of medical images are of the same interest as in art-historical research: the history and the change of media in medicine are focuses, together with ethical concerns pertaining to the medical use of images and the generation and concept of human.

The second part is the relationship between the image and body and between image and knowledge. At the Klinik für Orthopädie (Clinic for Orthopaedics) of the Universität Heidelberg, patients' expectations for the images, body perceptions, and relationships created by imaging will be examined, where relationship creation refers to the image as the 'third person' in the context of the physician and patient. The Kliniken für Neuroradiologie und Psychosomatik (Clinic for Neuroradiology and Psychosomatics) of the Technische Universität München will research the virtual reporting of organs and psychosocial pathogenesis. The relationship between image and knowledge includes questions about the normativity of and decision-making authority about medical images, as well as questions about epistemology (status of medicine) and ontology (status of images). In Munich, for example, the image as a communicative factor is of special interest; this concept includes the description of images and decision-making in clinical settings.

The concept of image as a communicative factor is the third part of the project and refers to the relationship between the image and society. This part is divided into 3 fields: image and language, image and culture, and image and public. Image and language is concerned with questions about the communication between physician and patient, the development of terminology (about symptoms), and the processes of diagnosis and therapy. In addition to the clinical cooperation partners, Munich and Heidelberg, the Institut für Arbeit und Technik Gelsenkirchen (Institute for Working and Technology) will research the sociology of images in medical and public contexts. This research will include, in addition to the topic of image and language, the relationship between image and culture and image and public. In the cultural context, the history of seeing as well as concepts of imagination, perception, and awareness of images in medicine will be researched. Questions about the sociology of the use (or competent use) of images and justification by images (e. g., in the context of health insurance) are part of the topic of image and society.

5. CONCLUSION

This short overview of the project demonstrates the connections between the main topics and the cooperation of the collaborating partners. It is important to emphasize the interdisciplinarity of the project: all of the results will be collected at workshops and seminars at the Kulturwissenschaftliches Institut in Essen, which is responsible for coordinating the project. Additionally, postgraduate programs, study groups, and meetings with the cooperation partners in Munich and Heidelberg are planned, as is a presentation at the Museum Folkwang in Essen.

One goal of this project is to understand the technical imaging of medicine. We predict that the research on the relationships between image, body, and knowledge will demonstrate that there is a need for a genuine critical appraisal of medical images for the protection of humanity in modern image-based medicine.

6. REFERENCES

Adelmann, Ralf & Jan Frercks (eds) (2009) 'Datenbilder. Zur digitalen Bildpraxis in den Naturwissenschaften' (Bielefeld: Transcript).
Allegretti, Peter (2011) 'Your Body: in the Focus', Medical Solutions May 2011 (Siemens): 62–67.
Baudrillard, Jean (2000) 'Denn die Illusion steht nicht im Widerspruch zur Realität', in Belting, Hans & Dieter Kamper (eds), Der zweite Blick. Bildgeschichte und Bildreflexion (München: Fink): 263–272.
Belting, Hans (2001) ,Bild-Anthropologie. Entwürfe für eine Bildwissenschaft' (München: Fink).
Belting, Hans (2002) 'Menschenbild und Körperbild', Das Bild des Menschen in den Wissenschaften (Gerda Henkel Stiftung) (Münster: Rhema): 149–180.
Belting, Hans (2004) 'Echte Bilder und falsche Körper – Irrtümer über die Zukunft des Menschen', in: Maar, Christa & Hubert Burda (eds), Iconic turn. Die neue Macht der Bilder (Köln: Du Mont): 350–365.
Boehm, Gottfried (eds) (1994) ,Was ist ein Bild?' (München: Fink).
Boehm, Gottfried (2007) ,Wie Bilder Sinn erzeugen. Die Macht des Zeigens' (Berlin: University Press).
Bredekamp, Horst & Gabriele Werner (eds) (2003) ,Bildwelten des Wissens.' Kunsthistorisches Jahrbuch für Bildkritik 1(1).

Breidbach, Olaf (2000) *,Das Anschauliche oder über die Anschaulichkeit von Welt'* (Wien, New York: Springer).

Breidbach, Olaf (2005) *,Bilder des Wissen. Zur Kulturgeschichte der wissenschaftlichen Wahrnehmung'* (München: Fink).

Breidbach, Olaf (2006) *'Naturbilder und Bildmodelle. Zur Bildwelt der Wissenschaften'*, in: Hinterwaldner, Inge & Marcus Buschhaus (eds), *The Picture's Image. Wissenschaftliche Visualisierungen als Komposit* (München: Fink): 23–49.

Burri, Regula (2008) *'Doing Images. Zur Praxis medizinischer Bilder'* (Bielefeld: Transcript).

Canguilhem, Georges (1974) *'Das Normale und das Pathologische' (1943/1966)* (München: Hanser).

Daston, Lorraine & Peter Galison (2007) *'Objektivität'* (Frankfurt/M.: Suhrkamp).

Fleck, Ludwig (1983) *'Erfahrung und Tatsache. Gesammelte Aufsätze' (1927–1960)* (Frankfurt/M.: Suhrkamp).

Foucault, Michel (1971) *'Die Ordnung der Dinge. Eine Archäologie der Humanwissenschaften' (1966)* (Frankfurt/M.: Suhrkamp).

Foucault, Michel (1973) *'Die Geburt der Klinik. Eine Archäologie des ärztlichen Blicks' (1963)* (München: Hanser).

Habermas, Jürgen (2001) *'Auf dem Weg zu einer liberalen Eugenik? Der Streit um das ethische Selbstverständnis der Gattung.'*, in Habermas (eds), *Die Zukunft der menschlichen Natur. Auf dem Weg zu einer liberalen Eugenik?* (Frankfurt/M.: Suhrkamp): 43–125.

Hagner, Michael (1996) *'Der Geist bei der Arbeit. Überlegungen zur visuellen Repräsentation cerebraler Prozesse'*, in: Borck, Cornelius (eds), *Anatomien medizinischen Wissens. Medizin – Macht – Moleküle* (Frankfurt/M.: Fischer): 259–286.

Heidegger, Martin (1980) *'Die Zeit des Weltbildes (1938)'*, in: *Holzwege* (Frankfurt/M.: Klostermann): 73–110.

Heintz, Bettina & Jörg Huber (eds) (2001) *'Mit dem Auge denken. Strategien der Sichtbarmachung in wissenschaftlichen und virtuellen Welten'* (Wien, New York: Springer).

Heßler, Martina & Dieter Mersch (eds) (2009) *'Logik des Bildlichen. Zur Kritik der ikonischen Vernunf't* (Bielefeld: Transcript).

Jacobi, Rainer-M. E. (2008) *'Gegenseitigkeit und Normativität. Eine problemgeschichtliche Skizze zu den Grundfragen medizinischer Ethik'*, in: Gahl, Klaus & Peter Achilles & Rainer-M. E. Jacobi (eds), *Gegenseitigkeit. Grundfragen medizinischer Ethik* (Würzburg: Königshausen & Neumann): 461–492.

Merleau-Ponty, Maurice (1964) *'Das Sichtbare und das Unsichtbare'* (München: Fink).

Mitchell, William J. T. (eds) (1994) *'Picture Theory. Essays on Verbal and Visual Representation'* (Chicago: University Press).

Mitchell, William J. T. (2008) *'Bildtheorie'* (Frankfurt/M.: Suhrkamp).

Stahnisch, Frank & Heijko Bauer (eds) (2007) *'Bild und Gestalt: Wie formen Medienpraktiken das Wissen in Medizin und Humanwissenschaften?'* (Hamburg: LIT).

Weizsäcker, Viktor v. (1997) *'Der Gestaltkreis. Theorie der Einheit von Wahrnehmen und Bewegen (1940)'*, in: *Gesammelte Schriften 4* (Frankfurt/M.: Suhrkamp): 77–337.

Wiesing, Lambert (2005) *'Artifizielle Präsenz. Studien zur Philosophie des Bildes'* (Frankfurt/M.: Suhrkamp).

'SEHKOLLEKTIV':
SIGHT STYLES IN DIAGNOSTIC COMPUTED TOMOGRAPHY[1]

Kathrin Friedrich

ABSTRACT

This paper aims to trace individual as well as collective aspects of 'sight styles' in diagnostic computed tomography. Radiologists need to efficiently translate the visualized data from the living human body into a reliable and significant diagnosis. During this process their visual thinking and the created images are incorporated into a complex network of other visualizations, communication strategies, professional traditions, and (tacit) visual knowledge. To investigate the interplay of collective as well as individual dimensions of diagnostic seeing, the concept of 'sight collective' (*Sehkollektiv*) is developed. On the one hand, this concept is based on critical reading of Ludwik Fleck`s epistemological writings and his notions of thought collective (*Denkkollektiv*) and thought style (*Denkstil*). On the other hand, it is tested by means of qualitative empirical studies in a radiological university clinic (participatory observations and informal interviews). By employing this approach, the paper traces the collective foundations of a certain diagnostic sight. Moreover, it shows how the individual abilities of radiologists to perform stylized seeing rely remarkably on software-based interactions with the processed images and on tacit dimensions of visual knowledge.

COMPLEX PROCESSES:
VISIBILITY IN DIAGNOSTIC COMPUTED TOMOGRAPHY

Computed tomography $(CT)^2$ images unfold as a complex and intersected process of technological requirements, visual knowledge, and socio-cultural inscriptions. By focusing on the question how a specific way of diagnostic seeing is established and applied, this paper explores the collective as well as the individual aspects that constitute a certain 'sight collective'.

---

1   This paper also appeared in Medicine Studies 2010
2   In short, computed tomography is a medical imaging process that employs rotating X-rays to create a computer processed volume of data (tomograms). The data sets are usually displayed as grayscale visualizations of body slices that can be manipulated on the screen by software tools. For a socio-cultural history of the development of CT in the USA, see e. g., Holtzmann Kevles (1997, pp. 143–172) as well as on performing a CT scan Saunders (2008, pp. 93–129).

To develop the conceptual framework of sight collective I draw on Ludwik Fleck's ideas of thought collective and thought style, however, and extend them in a critical perspective to capture also the (tacit) individual skills that support the diagnostic sight.

This framework was inspired by (and at the same time reassessed by) participatory observations and informal interviews at a radiological department of a German university hospital.[3] There I observed the processes of image capturing by computed tomography and case-based diagnosing in an everyday work routine setting for 3 weeks. During the stay, questions as follows arose: Are the applied imaging modalities referring to a certain visual tradition? Which socially conditioned factors are constituting and influencing the diagnostic sight? And: How can tacit dimensions of visual knowledge be traced?

To grasp these issues as facets of what I would like to call sight collective (*Sehkollektiv*), I am referring to Ludwik Fleck but also to Michael Polanyi's ideas on the tacit dimensions of knowledge. By extending and altering Fleck's perspectives it is possible to expose the collective – i.e. educational, socio-cultural, and practiced – dynamics which establish the framework of individual diagnostic seeing and knowing within a community like a radiology department. Or, as a senior radiologist reported during diagnosing CT images: "We have a certain amount of optic experience. Sometimes I cannot say why something on the screen is a lesion and not an artefact, but it is – I just see it."[4]

'ELUSIVE FACTORS': EXPANDING FLECK'S EPISTEMOLOGY

"An 'empty mind' does not perceive, does not compare, does not supplement: does not think" (*Fleck 1986d [1936], p. 110*).

In order to detect the collective foundations and dynamics of CT diagnosing, I refer to the framework of Ludwik Fleck's epistemology of science and medicine. His writings offer valuable theoretical, since practice-grounded, explanations based on "an amalgam of philosophy, history, and sociology, [which] anticipated the naturalizing and historicizing tendencies of contemporary philosophy of science" (*Fagan 2009, p. 273*). The basic notions of his theory are thought collective and thought style, which are dynamic and relational visions to trace the socio-cultural and historical properties of scientific knowledge (*Fleck 1986d [1936], p. 79*). Fleck's "essentially interactive, social and developmental" (*Fagan 2009, p. 273*) epistemology is based on the observation of three fundamental phenomena.

First, the "collective mental differentiation of men" (*Fleck 1986d [1936], p. 81*) allows people to communicate and understand each other because they "think

---

3   For comprehensive ethnographic case studies of tomography in medical contexts, see e.g., Beaulieu (2001, 2002), Cohn (2004), and Dumit (2004) on neuroimaging; Burri (2008a), Joyce (2008), and Prasad (2005) on MRI; Barley (1984, 1986) and Saunders (2008) on CT.

4   All following quotes from radiologists of the observed radiological department are translated by the author.

somehow similarly" and belong "to the same thought group" (*Fleck 1986d [1936]*, *p. 81*). This thought group is what Fleck actually calls thought collective, a "community of persons mutually exchanging ideas or maintaining intellectual interactions" (*Fleck 1979, p. 39*). Here every act of knowing, i.e., also visual knowledge, relates to previous historical traditions, education, and training, which constitute a certain thought style that is constantly stabilized by thought constraint (*Denkzwang*) but also slightly transformed by communication of thoughts within and also among collectives (*Denkverkehr*) (*Fleck 1986d [1936], p. 103*).

The latter points to the second phenomenon, which is "the circulation of thought [that] is always related, in principle, to its transformation" (*Fleck 1986d [1936]*, *p. 85*). The circulation varies according to the different layers of a thought collective, namely esoteric and exoteric circles (*Fleck 1986d [1936], p. 103*), but also among thought collectives, although sometimes no communication is possible as their thought styles are fundamentally different.

The relevance, content, and structure of scientific knowledge (e. g., a certain anatomical understanding) are defined by the thought style and emerge from what Fleck calls proto-ideas (*Urideen*) (Brorson 2000; Rotenstreich 1986). This somewhat blurry term (*cf. Löwy 1988, p. 150*) frames the third fundamental phenomenon of Fleck`s epistemology, which is "the *existence of a specific historical development of thinking, which cannot be reduced to the logical development of thought-contents nor to the simple increase of detailed information.*" (*Fleck 1986d [1936], p. 89, italics in original*). According to Fleck, on a methodological level, historical situations could not be merely traced by contemporary empirical methods because they "*show a world which is completely strange for us but not without a specific style.* "(*Fleck 1986d [1936]*, *p. 89, italics in original*). He suggests conducting closer studies without applying contemporary thought styles by substituting "today's content for the words" (*[Fleck 1986d [1936], p. 91*). Instead, "two measures which are at the disposal of the scientific thought style for giving the character of things its creations" (*[Fleck 1986d [1936], p. 108*) are main starting points to investigate the "social nature of thinking and cognition" (*Fleck 1986d [1936], p. 98*). Those two measures are the development and use of technical terms as well as the scientific device and its application.

Furthermore, for the purpose of this paper, it is important to note the fundamental difference between medical and scientific cognition as stated by Fleck in his first epistemological essay on *Some Specific Features of the Medical Way of Thinking* (1927). Unlike a natural scientist, a "medical man studies precisely the atypical, abnormal, morbid phenomena" (*Fleck 1986a [1927], p. 39*), which then again need to be somehow categorized due to communicability and the forming of disease entities. Hence, "the fundamental problem of medical thinking" is to "find a law for irregular phenomena" (*Fleck 1986a [1927], p. 39*). Thus, a certain medical thought collective cannot necessarily be described statistically in terms of its standards or basic concepts, i.e., an apparently affirmed thought style, but in terms of its 'standards' in dealing with aberrances and uncertainty as well as its flexibility of standpoint and vision within the given thought style (*Cook 2009, p. 6*).

To address those issues and to investigate the development of thought styles, Fleck adopts the concept of "specific intuition" (*Fleck 1986a [1927], p. 40*) without detailing it any further. He admits that "there come into play many elusive – as far as logic is concerned – imponderable factors which enable one to foresee (in a way forebode!) the course of problems which determine the development of a given field of thought and create its style peculiar to the epoch" (*Fleck 1986a [1927]*, *p. 40*). The historical development of medicine in particular and its thought styles cannot be described as merely a "matter of time, technical possibilities and accident" (*Fleck 1986a [1927]*, *p. 40*). Medical thought collectives need to efficiently develop a holistic vision of disease entities according to the given case, patient, and clinical context, because in any medical problem "it becomes ever and ever necessary to alter the angle of vision, and to retreat from a consistent mental attitude" (*Fleck 1986a [1927]*, *p. 43*). The thought style is constituted and developed within this framework and in exchange with other thought collectives, but what remains is a personal skill of each physician to align an overall thought style with pathology. Physicians have to vary collective boundaries according to the overall medical purpose to efficiently, nevertheless accurately, diagnose on the basis of mostly non-statistical, since human, indications (*Curtis 2004, p. 225*). Hence, there are no 'empty minds' in medicine, but it is crucial to recognize that these minds are not only filled with collective infiltrations but are also dependent on and interchanging with individual capacities. Even though Fleck stresses this specific feature of the medical profession, he does not offer an elaborated idea on his remark of specific intuition.

Based on my observations in a radiological department, I propose to integrate these 'elusive factors' of the development and application of a thought style into the investigation. Thus, it seems possible to grasp the yet invisible since 'imponderable' factors of diagnosing in computed tomography. Before doing so, I trace the foundations of a radiological sight collective which mutually constitute, enable, and alter individual and also tacit applications of a given sight style.

SKILFUL VISIONS: A RADIOLOGICAL SIGHT COLLECTIVE
(*SEHKOLLEKTIV*)

"(…) one has first to learn to look in order to be able to see that which forms the basis of the given discipline" (*Fleck 1986c [1935], p. 60*).

By speaking of sight collective instead of thought collective I want to shift the focus of attention towards the visual layers of collective and individual detecting, thinking, and diagnosing in computed tomography.

This research perspective basically assumes that vision is of course not only a perceptual capacity (looking) but also involves and constructs a certain way to think (seeing).[5] Consequently, at least three basic presumptions about medical images and visual perception that make up seeing are implied here.

---

5   On the basic philosophical discussion about the coherence of thinking and seeing or 'visual thinking' cf. Rudolf Arnheim (1969, pp. 1–37).

First of all, medical images themselves need to be 'visualized'. That might sound paradox, but becomes crucial when referring to images that are digital data on an ontological basis such as computed tomography images.[6] Leaving aside that these data themselves rely on techniques which prefigure the later way of visualization, digital data itself is primarily invisible and thus needs a display, i. e., a screen surface to be accessible for visible perception and immediately amenable for the observer.[7]

Furthermore, images need to be 'visible' by following-up cultural, historical, scientific, and/or social conventions of visualization and vision (*Cartwright 1995; Curtis 2004; Holtzmann Kevles 1997; van Dijck 2005*). Thereby, it should be standardized what 'has to be seen' and the possibilities of what 'could be seen' are intended to be rejected.

This leads to the third assumption, which rather points to the observer and thus connects to the epistemology of Fleck. The observer needs to 'see' and not only to 'look' if he wants to detect any content and any evidence in the image. As Fleck notes, seeing demands "a readiness for stylized (that is directed and restricted) sensation" (*Fleck 1979, p. 84*). Furthermore, I would add, seeing requires not only this readiness but also the ability to 'process' images and even to 'resist' them. Processing includes the ability to relate and connect them to other images, cultural and historical traditions, as well as other types of reasoning and thinking (*e. g., Arnheim 1980*). Resisting images contains selective seeing and curtailing visual information, e. g., reading a case anamnesis before looking at earlier images. Furthermore, it involves reducing environmental factors of visual perception, e. g., dimming other light sources or avoiding auditory amenities and secondary communication.

Radiology is obviously one of the most visual branches of medicine (*Wood 1999, p. 1*), even though clinical medicine itself relies significantly on visual senses and reasoning (*Foucault 2003 [1963]*). As I will illustrate, the skill to diagnose in computed tomography is mainly acquired by (a) education through embodying anatomical knowledge and the readiness for directional perception, (b) training and experience, and (c) (tacit) knowledge to render data intrinsically visible. The interplays of these collective as well as personal factors constitute the sight style in a specific sight collective of radiology, which is in this case a part of the radiology department in a university hospital.

The fact that the empirical part of my investigation is about a university hospital is of considerable importance. Physicians in such a clinic are used to students or observers who attend their work, thus they usually communicate and explain what they are doing. This kind of performative act somewhat preforms what is important

---

6   In his study on image interpretation in MRI, Amit Prasad supposes to rather use the term *image data* instead of images because tomographical visualizations "conveniently slide between being data or images." (Prasad 205, p. 292). On the (mathematical) modes to capture and reconstruct *image data* by medical imaging techniques see for example Schinzel (2009).

7   The notions of (algorithmic) subface and (aesthetically amenable) surface of digital data are invented by Frieder Nake (2008, pp. 104–108). On numerical representation as one of the principles of new media see Lev Manovich (2001, pp. 27–30).

to be observed and what could be neglected. Furthermore, I would like to stress the fact that CT is only a part of the radiology department. As I have observed, every radiological imaging technique, e. g., magnetic resonance imaging (MRI), radiography or, of course, nuclear imaging, requires and creates different dynamics in clinical work routines even though the technological unit (the apparatus and its requirements) as well as visual appearance of the data sometimes might seem quite similar. What comes into play here might seem trivial but influences imaging and diagnosing evidently. A radiographer who has closer contact with the patients in the MRI unit told me about her experience that if there is a relaxed atmosphere amongst physicians and radiographers, patients tend to be less afraid of the loud and claustrophobic technique. To not confuse those even harder to detect social interactions and atmospheres in different sections of the radiological department, I decided to focus in particular on the work routines in the CT unit.[8]

'To see one first has to know': The Readiness to See, and Embodied Knowledge

Curricula of medical education lay the foundations for later stylized seeing and diagnosing in CT.[9] In this respect and with the assumption that "[t]*o see, one first has to know*, and then to know how, and to forget part of the knowledge" (*Fleck 1986e [1947], p. 134, italics in original*) two basic capacities within the medical thought collective are prefigured, namely the formation of a more general and directed readiness to see and the embodiment of anatomical knowledge. I am here again relating to participatory observations during introductory lectures for first-semester medical students as well as to e-learning resources for advanced students in the elective course radiology.

Medical students are introduced to the internal and broad 'picture' of the medical profession and a core "medical gaze" (*Foucault 2003 [1963], esp. pp. 131–152*) during their studies. By means of this "sacrament of initiation" (*Fleck 1986d [1936], p. 106*), the student gets to know the formal structures as well as the collective's very own 'atmosphere'. This interplay results in a "readiness for directed perception and assimilation" (*Fleck 1979, p. 44*). From this moment onwards the student is incorporated by the collective body that defines the relevant information, problems, and objects of investigation (*cf. Fleck 1986d [1936], pp. 106–107*). Moreover, the student needs to anticipate the current (more common) 'medical visual culture', which is also fundamental for entering a radiological sight collective.

The introduction to the more general medical visual culture, the overall way to see and perceive the human body, happens amongst others by studying anatomy

---

8   Burri (2008b) examines how radiologists in different radiological branches, communities, and countries constitute their professional and disciplinary identities through boundary work and the accumulation of symbolic capital.

9   Examples for the design of curricula in radiological education are provided by van Deven et al. (2010).

(*Gunderman and Wilson 2005, p. 745*). Along with the student's own capability and disposition to visually perceive, anatomical knowledge is acquired by learning on the basis of several aesthetical resources, which involve different types and techniques of media and also living and dead bodies (*van Dijck 2005, pp. 118–137*). Anatomical handbooks, charts, models, and simulations converge on a consensual thought, and for this reason, sight style. A thorax schematically looks similar throughout literature (*Buschhaus 2005; Stafford 1991*), medical taxonomy is established as a common standard, and computer simulations of the inner body also share a common visual culture (*Waldby 2000*), not only in regard to medical but also to popular ways of looking (*Fleck 1986e [1947], p. 147*).

In dissection classes, anatomy becomes even more vivid, because the learning process is assured not only by vision but also by haptic evidence and the need "to couple visual investigation with verbal interrogation and reflection" (*Fountain 2009*). The students' own bodies are sensually invaded by their 'matter of studying' since they can immediately touch, smell, and see anatomical structures. Kenny Fountain concludes from his ethnographic studies in an anatomical lab: "The student of anatomy, then, brings together observation (the act of looking), visual evidence (what one sees in the body), haptic experience (the act of touching), and an-atomical-medical knowledge (what one labels the body) to identify as anatomy those objects on display" (*Fountain 2009*). Fountain's observations point to a radiologist's statement in an informal interview. This younger radiologist reported to me that almost every time he detects a fracture onscreen this reminds him of the anatomical dissections he had to do during his studies because at that time he had a corpse with an arm fracture. His sensual experiences – whether haptic, visual, or also olfactory – return when he sees a fracture because he embodied[10] the unmediated knowledge of dissection, which is updated again and again.

With the educational and embodied knowledge of not only anatomy but also with a prefigured 'medical vision' the student who decides to become a radiologist learns to see, e. g., computed tomography visualizations.

'A CERTAIN KNACK':
TRAINING AND EXPERIENCE IN DIAGNOSTIC RADIOLOGY

Besides their overall medical education, skilled radiologists have to be trained and experienced in their very own profession to diagnose "quickly and definitely nevertheless sustainably" as an experienced senior radiologist told a younger assistant

---

10   Following up on Kenny Fountain's remarks, the use of the term 'embodiment' at this point involves three intermingled notions: (1) the student's own body as an acting, perceiving, and observing one (cf. Polanyi 1964, p. 59–65, 88–90), (2) the observed object's own materiality, which constitutes the 'concrete' matter of knowledge, and (3) in Fleck's view, the collective body which sanctions and frames the interplay of subject and object (Fleck 1986d [1947], p. 147). On further discussion of the notion of 'body' and 'embodiment' in medicine, see for example Leder (1984) and Mol (2002).

radiologist. In everyday work routines, not only the repeated applications of the sight style but also collective meetings assure constraint on sight.

If we assume with Fleck that a diagnosis is "the filling of a result into a system of distinct disease entities" (*Fleck 1986c [1935], p. 64*) then a radiologist needs to know at least two factors: first, the system of disease entities and second, the possible results, whereas both determine each other. A future radiologist learns about the system of disease entities as part of a broad and not only radiological thought collective during his education. The result itself has to be compiled according to the system in every single case and is prefigured by the anamnesis, the request of the attending physician and the sight style. To quote the senior physician again: "We have a certain amount of seeing experience, which helps us to detect certain forms. (…) But you only see what you know".

By speaking about the detection of 'certain forms', the senior radiologist draws on one of the internal elements of sight style and the deployment of visual expertise which is the perception of forms (*Gestaltsehen*)[11] (*Wood 1999, p. 2*). Ludwik Fleck merely implicitly mentions gestalt theory without stating his sources (*Löwy, p. 142; Cohen and Schnelle 1986, p. xxi*). In his 1947 published article *To Look, To See, To Know* he mentions gestalt principles such as figure-ground relation, proximity, or similarity (*cf. Fleck 1986e [1947], p. 130*). In his opinion, if one is not able to develop a skilled vision, an 'economical' way of stylized seeing, "we look but do not see, we look intently at too many details without grasping the observed form as a definite entirety." (*Fleck 1986e [1947], p. 130*). Therefore, in radiological training, gestalt theory is considered to be helpful because it provides a conceptual framework to educate and train novice radiologists (*Hillard et al. 1985; Koontz and Gunderman 2008; Kundel and Nodine 1983; Kundel et al. 1972*). In everyday radiological work routines, "such fundamental gestalt concepts as figure-ground relationships and a variety of 'grouping principles' (the laws of closure, proximity, similarity, common region, continuity, and symmetry) are ubiquitous (…)." (*Koontz and Gunderman 2008, p. 1156*).

During my field research, I observed the application of gestalt principles in several cases which rely on the application of digital media technology. An example for the relation of the 'whole and its particulars' is the rendering of a topogram in CT. A topogram usually is preliminary to a sequence of scans to allow an overview of e. g. the patient's thorax. An experienced radiologist performs a rapid global search to identify normal anatomic structures with doubtful variations before going

---

11 At this point, the use of the term gestalt (cf. Arnheim 1969; Koffka 1922; Wertheimer 1912) relates to the basic theoretical concept that a form or a pattern is more than its particulars (Breidbach and Jost 2006, p. 19). Thus, a whole can only be perceived by relating the particulars and to cognitively fill the 'gaps' between them by, in this case, the seeing of similarities to previous cases (Prasad 2005, p. 292) in comparison to other occasions where such a form was detected (e. g., in the anatomy class). It also means, e. g., that a radiologist can concentrate on a detail (e. g., a lesion) without losing sight of the form of the organ and otherwise overlook other malformations (Prasad 2005, p. 305).

into detail, i.e., before schematically seeking for pathologic abnormalities (*Koontz and Gunderman 2008, p. 1157*).

Moreover, stylized seeing and visual expertise not only involve the incorporation of collective (visual) knowledge but also the creation of a visual memory with mental 'pre-images'. Those need to be manageable, i.e., there has to be an "experience of seeing many thousands of radiologic patterns and synthesizing them into a coherent, organized, and searchable mental matrix of diagnostic meaning and pathologic features" (*Wood 1999, p. 1*). An experienced radiologist updates previous relevant cases again just as he or she reads the anamneses and clinical request of a current case. In my observations I quite often witnessed questions among colleagues in the CT unit like "Do you remember the case of that pneumothorax last year?" Just before the radiologist sees current tomograms he knows what is ought to be seen. In the course of long practice and within the radiologist's 'visual memory', visual patterns are unified "with valid information to be retrieved when needed" (*Wood 1999, p. 1*). That makes the process of diagnosing even faster because detecting abnormalities does not last as long as in cases where one does not know what to look at.

In the observed CT unit also a 'materialized visual memory' of a broader sight collective could be found. Right next to the desk with computer screens for diagnosing there was a shelf where radiological handbooks and textbooks were available. With the help of these, or by Internet search mainly assistant doctors with a short-time experience in CT reassured themselves of e.g., taxonomies or topologies of organ sections. How often this (analogue) information was accessed depended on the experience, i.e., the number of similar cases before, the radiologist's own capacities to remember and update knowledge, and also doubts about peculiar forms. This procedure of "cross-referencing with other diagnostic inputs" (*Prasad 2005, p. 296*) helps to negotiate uncertainty in diagnosing, whereas I believe that certainty has to be understood as the personal matching of sight style.

The need to displace uncertainty is also met by the more or less collective convention to note in the diagnostic report that something is not visible in the applied technique (*Prasad 2005, pp. 300–302*). This means for example that in CT a pathologic transformation could not be detected, whereas it might have been visible in magnet resonance imaging, which is more precise in displaying tissue structures.

Another way to simultaneously negotiate individual uncertainty and perceive collective forms as well as their pathological aberrances is the schematic procedure of detecting, i.e., the technique of this particular sight collective to 'execute' diagnostic seeing. Not only does one of the decisive working principles in this sight collective, namely the procedure of 'detect-describe-diagnosis-document-discuss-differentiate' remain the same but also the way the process of detecting itself is structured. Hereby, the gestalt principles of similarity and symmetry are essential.

During my field research, an assistant radiologist was asked to diagnose the follow-up scan of lung cancer after therapy. To do this, he consulted the previous diagnosis and images, which lead his visual detection through "differential analysis" (*Prasad 2005, p. 292; see also Pasveer 1989, p. 367; Saunders 2008, p. 245*). In a first step, he aligned the current and previous images on both computer monitors by looking at similarities of the form of the lung region in case a different slice thickness or a different technique was used before. Then 'anchor points' were set by software applications in both image sequences to synchronize them and to assure visual orientation. Hence, it was possible to detect synchronously and symmetrically, i.e., in previous and current images at the same time, old lesions and, in comparison, look for new ones. The radiologist then 'traveled' through the lung on the axial plane from cranial looking at the left pulmonary lope on his way 'in' and at the right one when scrolling out. Thereby, he compared the older images with the new ones and looked for similarities of lesion affection. The procedure of visually detecting itself, i.e., the 'visual traveling through' the organs, remains the same according to the anatomical structure of the organ or region and case request. Besides, synchronously, a third screen displayed a standardized case protocol with prefigured text modules. On the basis of the anamnesis and diagnostic request of the actual case, the radiologist selected the protocol to guide the schematic procedure of his detection. Not only the topological structure but also the completeness of seeing is determined. Text modules, in addition to the above-mentioned global search, direct the seeing of certain forms in order to ensure time efficiency as well as completeness.[12]

Furthermore, guidance, but also control and constraint, in the observed sight collective are accomplished by collective meetings and the four-eye principle. The latter involves that every assistant doctor has to verify his diagnostic results with an experienced senior radiologist who visits regularly. Not surprisingly, he or she most often reads the diagnostic report before seeing the tomograms themselves. The assistant radiologist sometimes has to defend the diagnosis, i.e., his or her interpretation of the sight style in case the senior radiologist does not agree. In every discussion there is a learning effect and at the same time a sight restraint. By explaining the own diagnosis, the assistant radiologist reflects on his or her sight style and becomes more aware of pitfalls (*Atkinson 1995, pp. 73–89*). On the other hand, the experienced radiologist needs to mediate the collective sight style as well as his or her own meanderings within it. On an interpersonal level, negotiations about the 'right' way to see reflect the sight collective's own communication of sight and probably foreshadow forthcoming transformations (*Saunders 2008, p. 151*).

This restraint also occurs in the weekly department colloquia, where the director of the radiological department exemplifies certain cases. Everyone from a student in a practical course to an experienced senior physician has to prove his or her skills to see and not only to look, to answer questions and to listen to cross references of other cases. Sometimes external experts are invited to present new imaging

---

12 Timmermans and Berg argue that the construction and use of standardized (medical) protocols as means of *local universality* need to incorporate and transform routines and practices because this universality "rests on real-time work, and emerges from localized processes of negotiations and pre-existing institutional, infrastructural, and material relations." (Timmermans and Berg, 1997, p. 275) Therefore, they conceptualize a medical standard as "*a technoscientific script which crystallizes multiple trajectories*" (Timmermans and Berg, 1997, p. 275, italics in original).

techniques and to enable communication among other sight collectives. The style of seeing will not only be updated in everyday work routines, but it will also be brought in line in such collective meetings (*Saunders 2008, pp. 205–207*).

In summary, visual expertise or the 'certain knack' in CT diagnostics in this peculiar sight collective is achieved and assured by the perception of forms and schematic detection on several layers, internal and external visual memories as well as by collective meetings and interpersonal negotiations. Additionally, I want to trace the already mentioned 'elusive factors' or the tacit visual knowing, also in order to fill the 'gaps' of Fleck's epistemological ideas.

'I JUST SEE IT':
TACIT VISUAL KNOWLEDGE AND SOFTWARE INTERACTIONS

All of the features of diagnostic seeing in CT illustrated so far are more or less explicit, measurable, and analytically transferable. As outlined, a lot of this visual expertise relies on learning and training, but intermingled there is another quite important factor to explore the socio-cultural impacts on visual detection and reasoning, namely tacit knowing, i. e., the 'just' in the statement of the experienced senior radiologist: "Sometimes I cannot say why something on the screen is a lesion and not an artefact, but it is, I just see it."[13] Ludwik Fleck's above-mentioned hint on 'specific intuition' recalls indefinable and logically imponderable aspects of one's knowledge in contrast to statistics but he does not go into detail on this (*Fleck 1986a [1927], p. 40*).

In contrast, Michael Polanyi elaborated his theory of personal knowledge and tacit knowing[14] relying on medicine in his examples as well as in the use of transferred medical terms (*cf. Henry 2006, p. 191*). Polanyi's concept of tacit knowing is based on the assumption "*that we can know more than we can tell.*" (*Polanyi 1966, p. 4, italics in original*).

This tacit dimension covers intellectual as well as practical knowledge (*Polanyi 1966, p. 7*), which both depend on personal capacities in perception and awareness. Therefore, Polanyi synonymously uses the terms of skill and connoisseurship whereas the "medical diagnostician's skill is much an art of doing as it is an art of knowing." (*Polanyi 1964, p. 54*). Thus, for Polanyi, the body of a physician, like every human body, is "the ultimate instrument of all our knowledge" (*Polanyi 1966, p. 15*) as one dwells within it and acts from it. The body is the core of perception and also of action because it incorporates tacit knowing in the sense of 'thinking and doing', whereas visual perception presents "the main characteristics of a combined skilful knowing and doing" (*Polanyi 1961, p. 461*). In medicine, tacit knowing is mainly referred to as "the art of medicine" (*Malterud 2001, p. 398*),

---

13   The recognition of an artefact or *unidentified bright objects* as such influences amongst other factors whether the current health state is properly interpreted (Joyce 2005, pp. 450–452).

14   The use of the term 'knowing' instead of 'knowledge' relates to the dynamic character and practical aspects of implicit knowing.

which means that there has to be some kind of "skilful testing and expert observation, which cannot always be explicitly accounted for" (*Malterud 2001, p. 398*) to develop a reliable and also holistic diagnosis.[15]

During my field research, there was an occasion where the assistant radiologist who was on duty in the CT unit could not articulate what he was doing to diagnose. He used several software tools to alter the perspective of the currently displayed image sequences but he could not tell me why he did that action right at that moment: "I change the perspective, because then I can see better…But I do that almost every time when I am through the sequence and haven't found anything." Afterwards, his diagnosis corresponded with the one suggested by the experienced senior radiologist. Other assistant doctors who sometimes had to alter their diagnosis did not use the functions of the software tools and different image sequences as frequently and in such a wide range as he did.

Having observed this, I assume that the difference in stylized seeing as well as the tacit dimension of diagnosing relies largely on the radiologist's personal interactive use of the software tools in the picture archiving and communication system (PACS).[16] Here the graphical user interface (GUI) condenses intellectual and practical knowing because the handicraft of anatomical dissection is now accompanied by the 'sight craft' of digital imaging techniques. However, this is completed by a skill to act, precisely to interact with the software, and this interaction is mainly driven by the need to align images to sight style, to make data visible at the surface of the GUI.[17] Diagnostic seeing is in this case not only a collectively constituted mode of perception and knowing but also a skill and action to modify the object of investigation. "*To observe, to cognize (erkennen) is always to test and thus literally to change the object of investigation.*" (*Fleck 1986b [1929], p. 53, italics in original*). The instruments of dissections and the "mastery of tools" (*Polanyi 1961, p. 462*) become iconic represented algorithmic operations. Knowing not longer 'dwells' in the person's body alone, it emerges and becomes 'embodied' at the interplay of user and software technology.

A magnifier represented by a GUI has the same functionality as a magnifier for dissecting but its materiality is now substituted by the radiologist's own body, more

---

15 For instance, Maud Radstake`s ethnographic study shows how imaging by ultrasound and endoscopy mediates and transforms the perception as well as the body itself of both patient and physician (Radstake 2007).

16 Picture archiving and communication systems are provided by several health care companies to support "the storage, distribution, communication, display and procession of radiographic image data" (Tellioğlu and Wagner 2001, p. 163) within hospitals. One part of the network of a PACS is the graphical user interface within which digital data can be displayed, manipulated and compared to other (previous) images (Larsson et al. 2007; Tellioğlu and Wagner 2001).

17 This argument relates to Lev Manovich's remark that interaction is not only to be interpreted "literally, equating it with physical interaction between a user and a media object (…), at the expenses of psychological interaction. The psychological processes of filling-in, hypothesis formation, recall and identification (…) are mistakenly identified with an objectively existing structure of interactive links" (Manovich 2001, p. 57).

precisely by his or her index finger and visual system (*Alac 2008, 504*).[18] Sensual experiences such as the sense of touch or smell are transformed into the medical regime of visibility. Or to put it with the words of a senior advisor in radiology: "Clinical radiology is anatomy of the living subject."[19] Radiologists need to enter into 'strategic alliances' with the software in order to render the human body visually detectable[20], to combine particulars to create a familiar form (*Polanyi 1961, p. 463*). The reason for this is that they are faced with the problem of 'not seeing anything' if stylized seeing is too rigorously retained, whereas the prefigured knowledge of the anamnesis forces them 'to see something'.

Fleck, like Polanyi, also mentions the importance of instruments, tools, and apparatuses: "The scientific apparatus directs thinking towards the path of the scientific style of thinking: it produces a readiness to see certain forms, while removing at the same time the possibility of seeing others" (*Fleck 1986e [1947], p. 144*) and "a scientific appliance, which is a realization of some result of a definite thought style, directs our thinking automatically on to the tracks of that style" (*Fleck 1986d [1936], p. 109*). Consequently, in the observed operations in computed tomography, two 'instruments' of sight style interact, i. e., the radiologist's body as an incorporation and actor with a certain "style of action" (*Doroszewski 2007, p. 220; see also Malterud 2001, p. 398*), and the imaging technique which is visually represented by the GUI. In this interplay, tacit knowing emerges at the intersections of the collective as well as individual dimensions of the sight style.

CONCLUSIONS

"'To see' means: to re-create a picture, at a suitable moment created by the mental collective to which one belongs" (*Fleck 1986c [1935], p. 78*) and to apply one's own tacit knowing to the collective's sight style. A sight collective in diagnostic computed tomography is not only constituted by people who share the same thought style or in this case sight style, it is embodied in and at the same time transformed by every individual who acts on it without always being able to impart this. Hence, a sight style is not only constituted by collective aspects such as education or training, but also by individual skills, which enable radiologists to literally 're-create' these facets and match them with their individual abilities of seeing. As outlined, the interaction of collective and individual aspects of a sight style becomes 'visible' on the aesthetical surface of the GUI that frames the radiologist's connection to medical visual traditions and skills but also complements his or her ability to 'create' visibility in a certain case.

---

18 Alac (2008) explores the 'embodied actions' of neuroscientists while reading experimental data in form of fMRI images.
19 See also Kelly Joyce's ethnographic study on medical narratives about magnetic resonance imaging (Joyce 2005, p. 444).
20 On *rendering practices* deployed by natural scientists to transform the object's materiality into *docile objects* as scientific images see further Lynch (1985).

By exceeding and shifting Fleck's ideas, the concept of sight collective provides a tool to grasp also the individual and tacit aspects of sight styles. Certainly, this needs further qualitative research, in particular on the design of diagnostic software and human-computer interaction in radiology. As proposed for example by Paul Dourish, also "the interaction between the designer and the user *through* the system" (*Dourish 2001, p. 56, italics in original*) could be explored. If the designer "must structure the system so that it can be understood by the user, and so that the user could be led through a sequence of actions to achieve some end result" (*Dourish 2001, p. 56*), how much does the designer have to know about the user's sight style? This leads to issues of communication of sight among collectives, and additionally points to the question whether a tacit 'sight craft' could be anticipated or stimulated within a GUI.

REFERENCES

Alac, M. 2008. Working with brain scans. Digital images and gestural interaction in fMRI laboratory. *Social Studies of Science* 38(4): 483–508.

Arnheim, R. 1969. *Visual thinking*. Berkeley: University of California Press.

Arnheim, R. 1980. A plea for visual thinking. *Critical Inquiry* 6(3): 489–497.

Atkinson, P. 1995. *Medical talk and medical work. The liturgy of the clinic*. London: Sage Publications.

Barley, S.R. 1984. *The professional, the semi-professional, and the machines. The social ramifications of computer based imaging in radiology*. PhD dissertation, http://dspace.mit.edu/handle/1721.1/15401 (last accessed August 2010).

Barley, S.R. 1986. Technology as an occasion for structuring. Evidence from observation of CT scanners and the social order of radiology departments. *Administrative Science Quarterly* 31: 78–108.

Beaulieu, A. 2001. Voxels in the brain. Neuroscience, informatics and changing notions of objectivity. *Social Studies of Science* 31(5): 635–680.

Beaulieu, A. 2002. Images are not the (only) truth. Brain mapping, visual knowledge and iconoclasm. *Science, Technology and Human Values* 27(1): 53–86.

Breidbach, O. and J. Jost. 2006. On the gestalt concept. *Theory in Biosciences* 125: 19–36.

Brorson, S. 2000. Ludwik Fleck on proto-ideas in medicine. *Medicine, Health Care and Philosophy* 3: 147–152.

Burri, R.V. 2008a. *Doing images. Zur Praxis medizinischer Bilder*. Bielefeld: Transcript.

Burri, R.V. 2008b. Doing distinctions. Boundary work and symbolic capital in radiology. *Social Studies of Science* 38(1): 35–62.

Buschhaus, M. 2005. *Über den Körper im Bilde sein. Eine Medienarchäologie anatomischen Wissens*. Bielefeld: Transcript.

Cartwright, L. 1995. *Screening the body. Tracing medicine's visual culture*. Minneapolis: University of Minnesota.

Cohen, R.S. and T. Schnelle. 1986. Introduction. In *Cognition and fact. Materials on Ludwik Fleck*, ed. R.S. Cohen, and T. Schnelle, ix–xxxiii. Dordrecht: Reidel Publishing.

Cohn, S. 2004. Increasing resolution, intensifying ambiguity: An ethnographic account of seeing life in brain scans. *Economy and Society* 33(1): 52–76.

Cook, C. 2009. Is clinical gestalt good enough? *Journal of Manual and Manipulative Therapy* 17(1): 6–7.

Curtis, S. 2004. Still/moving. Digital imaging and medical hermeneutics. In *Memory Bytes. History, Technology, and Culture*, ed. L. Rabinovitz, and A. Geil, Durham: Duke University Press: 218–254.

Doroszewski, J. 2007. A methodological discussion of Ludwik Fleck's concepts of thought collective and thought style. In *Von der wissenschaftlichen Tatsache zur Wissensproduktion. Ludwik Fleck und seine Bedeutung für die Wissenschaft und Praxis*, ed. B. Choluj, and J.C. Joerden, Frankfurt/Main: Peter Lang: 213–237.

Dourish, P. 2001. *Where the action is. The foundations of embodied interaction*. Cambridge: MIT Press.

Dumit, J. 2004. *Picturing personhood. Brain scans and biomedical identity*. Princeton: Princeton University Press.

Fagan, M.B. 2009. Fleck and the social constitution of scientific objectivity. *Studies in History and Philosophy of Biological and Biomedical Sciences* 40: 272–285.

Fleck, L. 1979. *Genesis and development of a scientific fact*. Chicago: University of Chicago Press.

Fleck, L. 1986a [1927]. Some specific features of the medical way of thinking. In *Cognition and fact. Materials on Ludwik Fleck*, ed. R.S. Cohen and T. Schnelle, Dordrecht: Reidel Publishing: 39–47.

Fleck, L. 1986b [1929]. On the crisis of reality. In *Cognition and fact. Materials on Ludwik Fleck*, ed. R.S. Cohen and T. Schnelle, Dordrecht: Reidel Publishing: 47–59.

Fleck, L. 1986c [1935]. Scientific observation and perception in general. In *Cognition and fact. Materials on Ludwik Fleck*, ed. R.S. Cohen and T. Schnelle, Dordrecht: Reidel Publishing: 59–79.

Fleck, L. 1986d [1936]. The problem of epistemology. In *Cognition and fact. Materials on Ludwik Fleck*, ed. R.S. Cohen and T. Schnelle, Dordrecht: Reidel Publishing: 79–113.

Fleck, L. 1986e [1947]. To look. To see. To know. In *Cognition and fact. Materials on Ludwik Fleck*, ed. R.S. Cohen and T. Schnelle, Dordrecht: Reidel Publishing: 129–153.

Foucault, M. 2003 [1963]. *The birth of the clinic*. London: Routledge Classics.

Fountain, T.K. 2009. Anatomy education and the observational-embodied look. *Medicine Studies*. DOI 10.1007/s12376-010-0040-6

Gunderman, R.B., and Ph.K. Wilson. 2005. Exploring the human interior. The roles of cadaver dissection and radiologic imaging in teaching anatomy. *Academic Medicine* 80(8): 745–749.

Henry, S.G. 2006. Recognizing tacit knowledge in medical epistemology. *Theoretical Medicine and Bioethics* 27: 187–213.

Hillard, A., M. Myles-Worsles, W. Johnston, and B. Baxter. 1985. The developmet of radiological schemata through training and experience. A preliminary communication. *Investigative Radiology* 20: 422–425.

Holtzmann Kevles, B. 1997. *Naked to the bone. Medical imaging in the twentieth century*. New York: Basic Books.

Joyce, K.A. 2005. Appealing images. Magnetic resonance imaging and the production of authoritative knowledge. *Social Studies of Science* 35(3): 437–462.

Joyce, K.A. 2008. *Magnetic appeal. MRI and the myth of transparency*. Ithaca: Cornell University Press.

Koffka, K. 1922. Perception. An introduction to gestalt theory. *Psychological Bulletin* 19(10): 531–581.

Koontz, N.A., and R.B. Gunderman. 2008. Gestalt theory. Implications for radiology education. *American Journal of Roentgenology* 190: 1156–1160.

Kundel, H.L., and C.F. Nodine. 1983. A visual concept shapes image perception. *Radiology* 146: 363–368.

Kundel, H.L., and P.S. La Folette Jr., 1972. Visual search patterns and experience with radiological images. *Radiology* 103: 523–528.

Larsson, W., P. Aspelin, M. Bergquist, K. Hillergård, B. Jacobsson, L. Lindsköld, J. Wallberg and N. Lundberg. 2007. The effects of PACS on radiographer's work practice. *Radiography* 13: 235–240.

Leder, D. 1984. Medicine and paradigms of embodiment. *Journal of Medicine and Philosophy* 9: 29–43.

Löwy, I. 1988. Ludwik Fleck on the social construction of medical knowledge. *Sociology of Health and Illness* 10(2): 133–155.

Lynch, M. 1985. Discipline and the material form of images. An analysis of scientific visibility. *Social Studies of Science* 15(1): 37–66.

Malterud, K. 2001. The art and science of clinical knowledge. Evidence beyond measures and numbers. *Lancet* 358: 397–400.

Manovich, L. 2001. *The language of new media*. Cambridge: MIT Press.

Mol, A. 2002. *The body multiple: Ontology in medical practice*. Durham: Duke University Press.

Nake, F. 2008. Surface, interface, subface. Three cases of interaction and one concept. In *Paradoxes of interactivity. Perspectives for media theory, human–computer interaction, and artistic investigations*, ed. U. Seifert, J. H. Kim and A. Moore, Bielefeld: Transcript: 92–109.

Pasveer, B. 1989. Knowledge of shadows. The introduction of x-rays in medicine. *Sociology of Health and Illness* 11(4): 360–381.

Polanyi, M. 1961. Knowing and being. *Mind* 70(280): 458–470.

Polanyi, M. 1964. *Personal knowledge. Towards a post-critical philosophy*. New York: Harper Torchbooks.

Polanyi, M. 1966. *The tacit dimension*. Garden City, New York: Doubleday and Company.

Prasad, A. 2005. Making images/making bodies. Visibilizing and disciplining through magnetic resonance imaging (MRI). *Science, Technology, and Human Values* 30(2): 291–316.

Radstake, M. 2007. *Visions of illness. An endography of real-time medical imaging*. Delft: Eburon.

Rotenstreich, N. 1986. The proto-ideas and their aftermath. In *Cognition and fact. Materials on Ludwik Fleck*, ed. R. S. Cohen, and T. Schnelle, Dordrecht: Reidel Publishing: 161–179.

Saunders, B. F. 2008. *CT suite. The work of diagnosis in the age of non-invasive cutting*. Durham/London: Duke University Press.

Schinzel, B. 2009. Recognisability and visual evidence in medical imaging versus scientific objectivity. In *Dynamics and performativity of imagination. The image between the visible and the invisible*, ed. B. Hüppauf, and Ch. Wulf, New York: Routledge: 339–357.

Stafford, B. 1991. *Body Criticism. Imaging the unseen in enlightenment art and medicine*. Cambridge, MA and London: MIT Press.

Tellioğlu, H., and I. Wagner. 2001. Work practices surrounding PACS. The politics of space in hospitals. *Computer Supported Cooperative Work* 10: 163–188.

Timmermans, S., and M. Berg. 1997. Standardization in action. Achieving local universality through medical protocols. *Social Studies of Science* 27: 273–305.

Van Deven, T., K. M. Hibbert, and R. K. Chhem. 2010. *The practice of radiology education. Challenges and trends*. Berlin, Heidelberg: Springer.

Van Dijck, J. 2005. *The transparent body. A cultural analysis of medical imaging*. Seattle: University of Washington Press.

Waldby, C. 2000. *The visible human project. Informatic bodies and posthuman medicine*. New York: Routledge.

Wertheimer, M. 1912. Experimentelle Studien über das Sehen von Bewegung. *Zeitschrift für Psychologie* 61: 161–265.

Wood, B. P. 1999. Visual Expertise. *Radiology* 211: 1–3.

IV. ETHICAL CONSIDERATIONS

LOOKING BEHIND THE IMAGE: PHILOSOPHICAL AND ETHICAL ISSUES IN MEDICAL IMAGING

Santiago Sia

ABSTRACT

The ethical issue of justification has become an urgent challenge in medical imaging. There has been a shift in emphasis in the discussion: from what has been regarded as a rather paternalistic attitude of practitioners to one which stresses the rights of the individual patients. Since my contribution is meant to be a philosophical one, rather than scientific or medical, my concern here is to reflect on this current move on the part of the profession by offering certain philosophical considerations which are relevant to the present discussion on this topic.

I will discuss what is involved in the ethical task and its challenges and in the search for ethical justification. My main aim in this paper is to remind us of the need, and to stress the importance, of 'looking behind the image' by examining closely some of the ethical issues which arise from the practice of medical imaging.

INTRODUCTION

There has been some move on the part of the medical and scientific professions to focus on the issue of justification as it applies to them (Malone 2008).[1] This gathering, as well as similar ones in the past, attests to this. The move appears to be in the form of a shift in emphasis: from what has been regarded as a rather paternalistic attitude of practitioners to one which stresses the rights of the individual patients. There are several implications, some of which have already been noted elsewhere (Wikman-Svahn, n. d.) (Hansson 2007) (Binchy 2008).[2] Since my contribution to

---

1   Jim Malone, in 'New Ethical Issues for Radiation Protection in Diagnostic Radiology', refers to the need for the development of what he calls the fundamental ethical basis for the practices in radiology given a period of changing social attitudes. Reporting on the SENTINEL Dublin Workshop, he identified, among others, several ethical issues revolving around justification which arose in the discussions but which deserve further consideration. In this context, he welcomes the contribution that a philosophical perspective can make to the discussions, noting that such a contribution would take the form of identifying and articulating the arguments for and against particular ethical positions. Cf. J. F. Malone (ed.), *Proceedings of the Workshop on Radiation Protection in Medicine*. Special Issue of *Radiot. Protect. Dos* (2008).

2   In his paper 'The Ethical Foundation of Radiation Protection – from Utilitarianism to an Individual-oriented Philosophy' Per Wikman-Svahn observes that present radiation practices are essentially based on the application of the ALARA principle, which he maintains is commonly

this conference is meant to be a philosophical one, rather than scientific or medical, my concern here is to reflect on this current move on the part of the professions by offering certain ethical considerations which are relevant to the present discussion on this topic. My main aim is to encourage us to 'look behind the image', as it were.

SOME CLARIFICATIONS REGARDING ETHICS

But let me, at the outset, introduce some clarification regarding ethics itself. The first point that I want to state and clarify is that ethics and ethical conduct are much more than merely following an agreed way of behaving – the impression one gets from all the talk about the need for ethics in various areas or fields. Having a code of conduct is of course important and essential, but it would be misleading to think that 'ethics' or 'ethical decision/judgment' is merely a matter of 'going by the book', as it were. That is what makes discussions regarding ethical issues, be they in radiology or in any other areas, so complicated and so seemingly inconclusive.

believed to be founded on the ethical tradition of utilitarianism. Commenting on the approach taken by ICRP, he writes further that the proposed changes to the radiation protection system shifts the emphasis from the ALARA-principle to a principle of individual exposure-limitation. This means, in his view, that the ethical discussion moves more to a consideration of the rights of the individual. Cf. Feltz and Eggermont (eds.), *Ethics and Radiological Protection* (Louvain-la-Neuve: Academia Bruylant, n. d.).

Sven Ove Hansson in 'Ethics and Radiation Protection' makes a similar observation. While admitting that radiological protection and moral philosophy differ in many respects, he nevertheless claims an important and mutually beneficial dialogue that could exist between these two disciplines. He advances the view that 'some of the major problems in radiation protection are strongly connected with those that moral philosophers have worked with since antiquity.' He singles out what he calls 'the problem of combining respect for individual rights with the furthering of collective interests'. *Journal of Radiological Protection,* 27 (2007), 147–156.

Addressing the subject of justification of medical exposure, William Binchy notes that the *Medical Exposure Directive* assigns a prominent place to this issue. Furthermore, he observes that this document directs us to the broader philosophical, ethical and social contexts of the discussion on justification. Turning to the justification principle, he focuses on the term 'a sufficient net benefit' used in this document. He explains that this criterion attempts 'to weigh the total potential diagnostic or therapeutic benefits to the individual and to society against the possible individual detriment to the individual while taking into account the alternatives'. He compares this criterion to the 'felicific calculus' of utilitarianism 'in which individual welfare is subsumed into a social calculation and in which the language of individual rights that are capable of withstanding social convenience is anathema.' According to Binchy, the Directive does not adopt any particular philosophy in this context nor provide specific guidance on what outcome one is to expect. While appreciating the problematic situation that the Directive finds itself in, Binchy nonetheless faults the language of the Directive for not making overt reference to the concepts of human dignity, autonomy and bodily integrity. He would have liked the document to have acknowledged the complexity of the problem and the difference 'between balancing benefits against detriment in respect of one particular person and balancing social benefits against one particular person's detriment', adding that these two questions raise quite different issues. 'Justification of Medical Exposures and Medico-legal Exposures,' http://ec.europa.edu/energy/nuclear/radioprotection/publication/doc/102_en.pdf.

Why? Because when we ask what the ethical thing to do is in a situation, it is a question that is actually multi-faceted. It is not the same as merely asking for information, as when we ask for directions to reach our destination. In ethical discourse, for instance, asking the question: 'How much radiation would be considered ethical?' or 'Should one risk yet another exposure to radiation?', we need to consider not just what it is that we are proposing to do, but also why we want to do it, how it would affect various parties, whether this is in keeping with values that we ought to uphold, whether we are setting precedents, or whether we would be acting if there were the risk that everyone else would be following our example. Acting ethically, whether personally or professionally is much more complex and involved than simply adopting a code of conduct or following certain agreed guidelines.

My first point leads me to the second, and here I want to single out the ethical debate in scientific or medical circles, including this gathering. The kind of questions that drives our interests in these fields and those that need to be pursued in ethics are quite distinct. Scientific and medical endeavours, as I understand them, are not only largely based on what is tangible, what can be verified, but also and perhaps more importantly, on what can be done. Science or medicine concerns itself with pushing the boundaries of what we presently know about ourselves and the world we live in. Not only is this a legitimate enterprise, it is also in many ways one that has developed and even improved our lives. Ethics, for its part, is about what we ought to do or not do. And in many cases, what we can do, what we want to do, what we are told to do – is something different from what we ought to do. It is therefore a different line of inquiry compared to the scientific or medical one, but just as legitimate.

Does this mean then that ethical considerations always set limits to what we can do? Does this amount to saying that science or medicine and ethics are poles apart? Should we call a halt now to genetic testing, to stem cell research, or to our use of radiation, because it may be deemed unethical? Not necessarily. First, because both questions: 'What can we do?' and 'What ought we to do?' are important *human* questions. It is the same humanity that enables scientists, medical experts, and ethicists to ask and to pursue those questions. Secondly, what this means is that we cannot or ought not to totally exclude either question from our considerations. As we seek, in science or medicine, to enlarge our knowledge and our capabilities, or as we pursue greater control of our destiny, we also need to pause and ask: 'Ought we to go any further?' Similarly, those of us who are more concerned with the ethical question, 'Ought we to do or not do it?' should also stop and ask ourselves: 'What can we do further?' What this last comment means for ethicists is that ethics and ethical decision-making cannot simply be informed by past knowledge or by moral principles that we have worked out based on information available then. We also have to listen to and be informed by developments in empirical science even to the extent of revising our ethical judgments.[3] Why? Because even if we can defend

---

3   The issue of ethical relativism comes to mind here. If by relativism is meant the philosophical doctrine which maintains that everything is relative, then clearly this would be contradictory since even that statement that everything is relative is itself relative and therefore need not be

the view that there are moral absolutes, our knowledge of what is ethical in specific matters is not absolute. The principles of doing good and avoiding evil at all times or of not inflicting harm on an innocent party are universally acknowledged, but how these principles apply to specific cases requires a more nuanced judgment. This is because application is always to specific cases or situations, and this move to the concrete situation from the abstract principle is dependent on several factors – some of which I had mentioned earlier. Developments in science and medicine are a prime example of this. They alert us to the need for ethicists to take account of the findings of these fields before making ethical judgments.

The ethical task, thus – in the present context, the search for an ethical criterion to justify the practice – is much more challenging in that it is rather complex because it involves so many factors. This is true in any professional context as it is in daily life. And yet one is expected to act – and to act ethically – despite this complexity. But this is really the nature of the ethical task: it is ultimately a human *judgment* on the part of the agent (that is to say, the 'doer of the action'). At the same time, however – and this is a crucial consideration, contrary to the views of many – the judgement made by the agent is not merely a completely subjective or arbitrary one. It is based on a *criterion* that has been seriously and fundamentally considered (that is to say, an ethical norm rather than a scientific fact). For this reason, the discussion on justification differs from the related discussion by this grouping that deals with the issue of optimization. We need to consider not just the action itself but also the nature of the agent and of the recipient of the action (Sia 2009).[4]

AUTONOMY AND CONSENT OF THE RECIPIENT

Let me now look even more closely 'behind the image' by addressing specific issues regarding justification and commenting on the shift in emphasis away from the agent towards the recipient of the act. This strategy brings to close range some important and fundamental philosophical issues such as the autonomy and the rights of the patient as well as the question of consent on the patient's part.

The current focus on the human individual's autonomy – even in contemporary philosophical thinking – is actually rooted in a long tradition that claims that each and every human individual is, to use Immanuel Kant's terminology, an 'end to itself'. This means that the individual's ability to exercise his or her freedom comes from within oneself, rather than from outside. It is therefore not conferred but acknowledged, and is, to adopt business-speak, non-negotiable. It is the basis for the fundamental rights of the individual that all others have a duty to respect. It is for

accepted as true. What is meant here rather is that in moral decision-making there is a certain amount of relativity not only because several subjective factors do influence our knowledge of what is right (or wrong) but also because ethical judgment must take into account the particularity of situations.

4   See my 'Justification and Radiology: Some Ethical Considerations,' *Radiation Protection Dosimetry,* http://rpd.oxfordjournals.org/cgi/reprint/ncp041

this reason that, as Kant would put it, every human individual has dignity and not just value.[5] Unlike the worth of a work of art or a material possession,[6] it is invariable and cannot be taken away without doing an injustice to that human individual. For Kant (and for the vast majority of philosophers) the human individual is therefore itself the source of one's law, and therefore is truly free and has inalienable rights. This autonomy is what identifies the human individual from every other creature. And this is, I believe, what underpins the shift in the justification debate in the professions towards the rights of the patient.

But the affirmation of human autonomy is complicated by the fact that such an exercise of freedom takes place within a social context. In other words, since every human individual is autonomous and since every such individual needs to exercise that autonomy within human society, a conflict of rights occurs when another person's rights are in opposition. There is a fundamental need to recognise and acknowledge that other human individuals are themselves centres of autonomy whose rights must also be respected. It is for this reason that Kant's view has been modified by others. The suggestion has been made that one must not regard human autonomy or human rights in absolute terms but that these rights should be prioritised. However, this is much more than just putting rights on a sliding scale – an impossible task in itself – but rather of putting the onus on those who wish to override the fundamental status and rights of the human individual to provide reasons which can legitimately and justifiably be accepted. In other words, the autonomy of the human individual remains intact *until* and *unless* there are good and solid reasons to affirm otherwise. In the case of an individual who is not in a position to exercise his or her autonomy, provisions must be made that still respect that individual's dignity. What these provisions are will depend on the particular situation.

To a large extent, this is where utilitarianism, particularly as developed by the philosopher JS Mill and nuanced by a number of contemporary philosophers, can be helpful in that it does supply us with a way towards reconciling competing claims by taking the consequences of one's action into consideration. Compared to the Kantian view, the need to reckon with the consequences – benefits and risks in the present context[7] – of our actions and to evaluate them in terms of the kind of impact and the number of affected parties gives a more tangible and manageable approach. The A.L.A.R.A. principle adopted in radiology has that advantage. However, it should be added that among others, the philosophical ethical theory of utilitarianism has also been criticised for sacrificing the individual good – and not always in a laudable way – by pushing forward what some may claim to be the

5   Some contemporary philosophers have introduced in their ethical discussion the distinction between the concept of 'human being' (a descriptive term) and that of the 'person' (a prescriptive term). The latter term implies a certain moral attitude or response on our part.

6   Given the present economic situation in the world, a more relevant comparison would be shares, stocks or pension funds!

7   The accepted phrase in radiology seems to be 'benefits and risks'. Strictly speaking, however, if one were referring to consequences, it should be 'benefit and harm (including possible harm)'. This is because taking risks itself can be justified since it is necessary for our development as human beings.

common good. Moreover, it can be accused – at least, in certain versions of utilitarianism – of prejudging both the kind and the extent of the consequences while ignoring the basic rights.

This philosophical discussion, despite its seemingly theoretical air about it, has practical implications, not least for our present context. The move in radiological practice towards affirming the patient's autonomy is in fact a recognition of the dignity of every patient as subject, rather than, object. In other words, the patient is not a thing to be worked on but rather is a unique individual. For this reason, the recipient of one's action is not a receiver of one's action in the same way as is an object in an assembly line is but instead requires individual personal attention.[8] Thus, the re-thinking of justification in radiological practice is not merely a move away from what was regarded as a paternalistic criterion but instead is an awareness of the status and the role of the recipient. In this context the solicitation of informed consent of the recipient is particularly relevant. What justifies the need for an informed consent is based on the nature of the recipient. As subject (in the ethical sense), that human individual must be respected as a human individual, and not merely the recipient of someone else's action. Informed consent is based on the individual's nature as a being with intellect and free will and so should be treated as such. Paternalism can be rightfully accused of promoting heteronomy – although it must be noted may not always be questionable in some cases, but is so in this instance – inasmuch as the decisions are being made on behalf of the recipient by others who believe that decision-making should be relegated to those who 'know best'; namely, themselves.

However, just as there are difficulties with the Kantian emphasis on the autonomy of the subject, we must also be aware that soliciting the consent of the recipient may not always nor necessarily be acting in their best interests as they may not understand the ramifications of the proposed action. The usual way of dealing with this issue is to turn to the phrase 'informed consent' or 'valid consent' (or to those who have been charged to act on their behalf). Having the relevant information regarding the action and communicating it to the recipient of the action is of course of primary importance in acknowledging the recipient as a human individual. As has been noted already, this is to acknowledge that he or she is entitled to such knowledge as befits his or her nature. But the situation is aggravated by the complexity of the data and the interpretation of the data. We have become aware of the enormity and complexity of the information that is thrust upon us by the increasingly rapid developments in today's scientific and technological world.

'Informed consent' should therefore not merely mean 'being in possession of the relevant information' but more crucially 'being able to process correctly all the information that has been given'.[9] This presents the agent of the action[10] with a dif-

---

8 A purely 'clinical approach' therefore ignores the humanity of the patient.
9 The issue of communication, already identified in the current discussion on justification in radiology, is particularly relevant. It is not simply 'imparting data' but dealing with a human situation.
10 The 'agent' is not merely as reference to the individual practitioner, but to the entire professional body. There is such a thing as 'collective responsibility'.

ficulty and may account for the paternalistic practice of withholding some information or of relegating decision-making to those who do have the expertise to make the right judgement. Worse, providing all the information to the recipient could lead to unacceptable consequences for the recipient, including damaging that individual's well-being.[11]

'Being able to correctly process all the information that has been given', therefore, means more than simply understanding the data but also means being able to correctly act on the data. This is where the 'consent' part of the phrase 'informed consent' is crucial. For 'consent' in the ethical sense – as distinguished from other contexts – is not simply agreeing on the basis of one's knowledge but also by 'being in a position to agree'. Such a situation differs from individual to individual and from case to case. Moreover, 'consent' refers to the recipient as one who has not just an intellect but also free will. This complicates the matter even further since the question could be asked as to how freely the consent was given. The patient may, in reality, be too ill to give consent. Outside pressures, in addition to circumstances, both individual and social, may limit the degree of freedom which an individual has to make decisions, including the decision to accept or reject medical treatment. The keyword in informed consent is 'voluntary'. Just as excluding the recipient from the decision process is ethically undesirable, in our attempts to re-think the ethical issue of justification in radiology, putting the onus of decision-making on patients may not always be the approach either if they are not in a position to really exercise their autonomy.

In the present context it is important therefore to keep in mind that what is really more crucial is not autonomy as such but *the exercise* of that autonomy. The distinction between the two is conceptual of course, and so somewhat abstract, but its reality is concrete and therefore has practical implications. So, while we must indeed respect the autonomous nature of each human individual, we must also be alerted to the actual situation when regarding its exercise. This is because the exercise of autonomy is always social: it is always over another. And that other, especially if it is also autonomous, has rights which must also be respected (Sia 2010).[12] And that is what leads sometimes to a conflict of rights, a situation which needs to be resolved. For this reason, the autonomy of the recipient cannot and should not be considered absolute. Otherwise, one could be accused of 'reverse paternalism' whereby we offload responsibility onto the recipient without considering if indeed the recipient – and I am not necessarily talking of extreme cases – is in a position to make a reasonable decision.

---

11   For this reason, clarity and accuracy of the communication are not sufficient as the human situation also calls for sensitivity on the part of the agent.

12   This point is particularly pertinent to specific cases like self-presentation, self-referral as well as the distribution of scant commodities. It also raises the issue of balancing public and individual interests. Cf. Chapter Seven of my *Ethical Contexts and Theoretical Issues: Essays in Ethical Thinking* (Cambridge Scholars Publishing, 2010).

THE MORAL SENSE OF THE AGENT

What has been described so far seems to be a return to, rather than a departure, from the agent in re-thinking the issue of justification. To a certain extent this is true but only because ethically, ultimate responsibility rests with the agent; that is, the doer of the action. However, it is not a simple return to the paternalistic attitude that has incurred some justified criticism and which has prompted this re-thinking. I am not advocating the claim that 'the practitioner knows best'; but rather, that the practitioner, who is the agent in this case, must ensure that he or she is acting from a sense of responsibility. Needless to say, that assumes the practitioner has the right knowledge base, i.e. being able to ascertain from a medical and scientific point of view that one has the most informed basis on which to act. If that knowledge is lacking, it would certainly be irresponsible for the practitioner to continue.[13]

Just as important in this context is the development what I call 'the moral sense of the agent'. Nurturing one's moral sense and applying it to all aspects of life is a difficult task, particularly when faced with new situations. Since moral judgements must sometimes be made, it is essential that we are guided by a moral sense that has been deepened and strengthened by continuous ethical reflections not only in day-to-day living but also in our professional endeavours. In this respect, the early education of practitioners in this area is truly crucial. Since practitioners deal with human subjects, they should understand the human situation and not simply the medical, clinical or technological side of their training.

Moral sense is much more than just moral sentiment or feeling. Nor is it an intuition or an intellectual ability that enables one to distinguish between right and wrong. Moreover, it is not simply a hunch that one follows when one exercises one's free will. And yet all of these come into play since moral sense is ultimately based on our very humanity.[14] As human beings, we possess feelings, intellect and free will, and when we ask what is ethical and what is not and draw a conclusion, we make use of all these gifts.

The word 'sense' carries different meanings, each of which we can avail of to shed light on 'moral sense' (as used in the present context). 'Sense', of course, means our five senses that enable us to be in contact with the outside world. The word is also used to refer to someone having 'sense'; and we mean that that person does not just know but has the right knowledge. It can also mean simply, 'in a particular instance', as when we qualify a statement or a claim when we say 'it is true in this sense'. But 'sense' can also have a stronger meaning as a more or less coherent overall view as when we talk of 'life making (or not making) sense'.[15]

---

13 In ethics, one talks not just of 'commission' but also of 'omission'. One is accountable not just for what one has done but also for what one should have done but has not done.

14 There is a close association of 'moral sense' with 'conscience', but I am distinguishing the two because certain connotations associated with one would not necessarily apply to the other.

15 Contemporary philosophy, influenced by the postmodern trend, has shied away from pursuing the so-called 'bigger picture' of life. However, there are signs that such a trend is being reversed.

The phrase 'moral sense' draws on these meanings. It is through our senses that we accumulate experience, including moral experience, of the world around us. We require the right knowledge, and not just any knowledge, to enable us to act ethically. We need to be aware of the particularity of a situation to enable us to judge the appropriateness of our judgement or decision. More importantly, we ought to be informed by an overall perspective that helps us not just to situate the particular moral situation or context but also to judge it more consistently.[16]

The various uses of 'sense' and their applicability to the phrase 'moral sense' means that ethics should not be interpreted as an instinctive, wilful or even a cerebral activity. It is a rational activity by which I mean that it involves all the abilities that human beings possess, including the use of our intellect.[17] And since it takes place in concrete situations and particular individuals, it is an activity that draws on various sources, including gender, culture and religion, and so on, whenever we resort to it.

Moral sense has a particular role to play in our ordinary and professional lives. The will to act must be spurred by our moral sense to ensure that we are indeed acting ethically. This is because the pursuit of ethics should lead not just to knowing what is right and wrong – in the broad sense indicated above – but ultimately to doing that which is right and avoiding that which is wrong. For this reason, there is a justified expectation that ethics should facilitate our becoming more responsible, more civic-minded, and better behaved. This is a greater challenge. On the other hand, while ethics itself may not necessarily lead to ethical conduct of the individual agent, it nevertheless promotes and sustains it, at least indirectly. While knowledge of what is right needs other factors to make us want and pursue the good, ignorance of relevant information, including what is involved in making the ethical judgement or decision can easily lead to irresponsible or unethical conduct. Since acting ethically is dependent on our knowledge of the situation, the more we know the relevant factors, including our moral norms, the less we are in danger of acting unethically.

In the decision-making process or the pursuit of an action, it is important to note that it is not simply a matter of deciding and then acting but of viewing the situation against a wider background. Situation ethics, which focuses almost exclusively on the particular situation or circumstance as dictating the morality of an action, ignores the need to be consistent in our ethical judgments. In ethics, what is appropriate or even what is legal is not only always the right ethical decision; and we should guard against making simply ad hoc decisions. In this respect developing a moral sense, defined as a sense of responsibility that is actuated by what we can do but is constantly guided by what we ought or ought not to do is particularly important. This underlies the need to view the larger picture and for teaching ethics as part of the medical school curriculum.

---

16 Contemporary ethical philosophers, like John Rawls in his *A Theory of Justice*, have moved away from pursuing merely metaethical issues to constructing ethical theories.

17 I am therefore distinguishing between 'reason' (usually associated with the use of the intellect) and 'rationality' (referring to the whole of human nature).

CONCLUDING COMMENTS

Acting ethically challenges us to provide a more consistent and more systematic answer to dilemmas. In some cases the answer to the question 'what ought I to do?' must be quick and even instinctive. But in the ethical context, one's answer should be much more thoughtful. This does not mean that every time we find ourselves with an ethical challenge, we cannot and should not act until we have undergone a prolonged and thorough process of thinking about the matter. Many cases, particularly medical ones, do not allow us that luxury for every problem. But the study of ethics in one's training and education in the professions can be of paramount importance as it can provide us with a 'theoretical framework' to enable an ethical solution to a problem. The basis for one's judgment, even those made in a hurry, may then be more firmly grounded. The purpose of an education in ethics is to expose underlying theoretical assumptions and subject them to a critical evaluation, and to provide an early warning system to potential problems in urgent cases. Ethics education helps to nurture one's moral sense by scrutinizing more critically not merely the question we are asking but also, and more importantly, the underlying assumptions behind those questions. The role of ethics is important in re-thinking the issue of ethical justification in radiology just as it is in every facet of life.

REFERENCES

Binchy, William (2008) *'Justification of Medical Exposures and Medico-legal Exposures'*, http:// ec.europa.edu/energy/nuclear/radioprotection/publication/doc/102_en.pdf

Hansson, Sven Ove (2007) *'Ethics and Radiation Protection'*, Journal of Radiological Protection, 27: 147–156.

Malone, Jim (2008) *'New Ethical Issues for Radiation Protection in Diagnostic Radiology'*, J.F. Malone (ed), Proceedings of the Workshop on Radiation Protection in Medicine. Special Issue of Radiot. Protect. Dos.

Sia, S. (2009) *'Justification and Radiology: Some Ethical Considerations'*, Radiation Protection Dosimetry, http://rpd.oxfordjournals.org/cgi/reprint/ncp041.

Sia, S. (2010) *'Ethical Contexts and Theoretical Issues: Essays in Ethical Thinking'* (Cambridge Scholars Publishing).

Wikman-Svahn, Per (n. d.) *'Radiation Protection – from Utilitarianism to an Individual-oriented Philosophy'* in Feltz and Eggermont (eds), Ethics and Radiological Protection (Louvain-la-Neuve: Academia Bruylant).

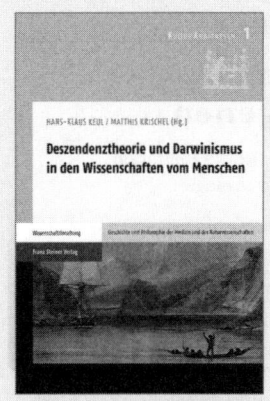

Franz Steiner Verlag

Hans-Klaus Keul / Matthis
Krischel (Hg.)
Deszendenztheorie und
Darwinismus in den
Wissenschaften vom Menschen

2011.
141 Seiten mit 11 Abbildungen.
Kart.
ISBN 978-3-515-09921-9

Hans-Klaus Keul /
Matthis Krischel (Hg.)

Deszendenztheorie und Darwinismus in den Wissenschaften vom Menschen

Kulturanamnesen – Band 1

Wie läßt sich Darwins Evolutionstheorie im Kontext
der Kultur der Moderne verorten? Die Beiträger
dieses Bandes widmen sich der Geschichte und
Bedeutung der Evolutionstheorie für die Humanwissenschaften, da hier Aspekte der natur- und
kulturwissenschaftlichen Entwicklungslehre mit-
einander verschränkt auftreten. Aus unterschiedli-
chen Perspektiven, etwa der Evolutionsbiologie, der
Philosophischen Anthropologie und Moralphiloso-
phie, der Psychologie, der Ethnologie und der
Theologie, erläutern die Autoren Facetten des
evolutionären Konzepts.
Doch geht es ihnen nicht um die Eröffnung einer
einheitlichen Perspektive auf die Entwicklung des
Menschen; wohl aber bieten die Beiträge
gemeinsam mit einer Themenvielfalt auch eine
Methodenvielfalt an und reflektieren kritisch auch
die Grenzen der jeweiligen Fachgebiete.

....

Die Herausgeber

Hans-Klaus Keul koordiniert an der Universität
Ulm das Ethisch-Philosophisches Grundlagen-
studium und den Bereich für additive Schlüssel-
qualifikationen.

Matthis Krischel ist wissenschaftlicher Mitarbeiter
am Institut für Geschichte, Theorie und Ethik der
Medizin an der Universität Ulm.

....

Franz Steiner Verlag
Birkenwaldstr. 44 · D – 70191 Stuttgart
Telefon: 0711 / 2582 – 0 · Fax: 0711 / 2582 – 390
E-Mail: service@steiner-verlag.de
Internet: www.steiner-verlag.de

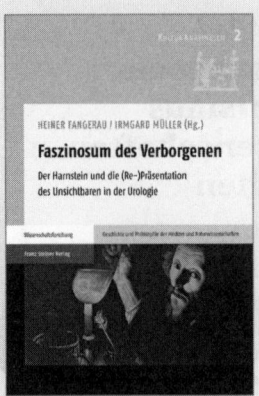

Franz Steiner Verlag

Heiner Fangerau /
Irmgard Müller (Hg.)
Faszinosum des Verborgenen

2012.
142 Seiten mit 50 Abbildungen.
Kart.
ISBN 978-3-515-10034-2

Heiner Fangerau /
Irmgard Müller (Hg.)

Faszinosum des Verborgenen

Der Harnstein und die (Re-)Präsentation
des Unsichtbaren in der Urologie

Kulturanamnesen – Band 2

Die (Re-)Präsentation des Unsichtbaren stellt ein
klassisches Problem der Medizin dar, das bis heute
nicht an Anziehungskraft verloren hat. Aus histori-
scher Perspektive lautet dabei eine der zentralen
Fragen, inwiefern sich Produktion und Darstellung
medizinischer Erkenntnis wechselseitig durchdrin-
gen. Gerade die urologische Technik, die zu den
ersten medizinischen Gegenstandsbereichen zählt,
die das Unanschauliche anschaulich gemacht
haben, bietet sich hier als Untersuchungsfeld an.
Nach einigen theoretischen Vorüberlegungen
werden in diesem Band Darstellungsformen von
Harnsteinen, die Bedingungen ihrer Sichtbarmachung und Entfernung sowie zuletzt ihre Reprä-
sentationsformen im therapeutischen Kontext
behandelt. Auf diese Weise wird die Vielfalt der
Ansätze zur Bildgenerierung und die Macht der
Bildproduktion an einem bisher in diesem Zusam-
menhang wenig beachteten pathologischen Objekt,
den Harnsteinen und ihrer versinnlichten Anschau-
ung, in Augenschein genommen und diskutiert.

....

Die Herausgeber

Heiner Fangerau ist Direktor des Institutes für
Geschichte, Theorie und Ethik der Medizin der
Universität Ulm.

Irmgard Müller war Leiterin des Instituts für
Geschichte der Medizin und Medizinhistorischen
Sammlung der Ruhr-Universität Bochum.

....

Franz Steiner Verlag
Birkenwaldstr. 44 · D – 70191 Stuttgart
Telefon: 0711 / 2582 – 0 · Fax: 0711 / 2582 – 390
E-Mail: service@steiner-verlag.de
Internet: www.steiner-verlag.de